Trauma Informed Care

Tamar Rodney
Editor

Trauma Informed Care

Practical Skills for Nurses

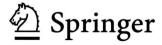

Editor
Tamar Rodney
Johns Hopkins University School of Nursing
Baltimore, MD, USA

ISBN 978-3-031-87525-0   ISBN 978-3-031-87526-7   (eBook)
https://doi.org/10.1007/978-3-031-87526-7

© The Editor(s) (if applicable) and The Author(s), under exclusive license to Springer Nature Switzerland AG 2025

This work is subject to copyright. All rights are solely and exclusively licensed by the Publisher, whether the whole or part of the material is concerned, specifically the rights of translation, reprinting, reuse of illustrations, recitation, broadcasting, reproduction on microfilms or in any other physical way, and transmission or information storage and retrieval, electronic adaptation, computer software, or by similar or dissimilar methodology now known or hereafter developed.
The use of general descriptive names, registered names, trademarks, service marks, etc. in this publication does not imply, even in the absence of a specific statement, that such names are exempt from the relevant protective laws and regulations and therefore free for general use.
The publisher, the authors and the editors are safe to assume that the advice and information in this book are believed to be true and accurate at the date of publication. Neither the publisher nor the authors or the editors give a warranty, expressed or implied, with respect to the material contained herein or for any errors or omissions that may have been made. The publisher remains neutral with regard to jurisdictional claims in published maps and institutional affiliations.

This Springer imprint is published by the registered company Springer Nature Switzerland AG
The registered company address is: Gewerbestrasse 11, 6330 Cham, Switzerland

If disposing of this product, please recycle the paper.

Preface

It is an honor to present *Trauma Informed Care*, a book that reflects the collective expertise, passion, and dedication of my colleagues, all of whom have worked extensively in the field of trauma. This book is the result of a shared commitment to providing better care for individuals affected by trauma, and I am deeply grateful to all those who contributed their knowledge and experiences to make this project a reality.

The aim of this book is to offer healthcare providers, particularly nurses, a comprehensive and practical guide for delivering trauma-informed care. Trauma is a complex, multilayered experience that affects individuals in ways that extend beyond physical injury, impacting emotional, mental, and behavioral health. As healthcare professionals, it is essential that we not only recognize trauma but also understand its far-reaching consequences so that we can address the whole person with empathy, understanding, and appropriate interventions.

The chapters in this book explore the acute and long-term effects of trauma, including post-traumatic stress disorder (PTSD), as well as the biological, behavioral, and generational dimensions of trauma. The contributors have provided invaluable insights into how trauma shapes not only the individual but also the communities and families around them, emphasizing the need for an informed, compassionate approach to care.

One of the unique aspects of this book is the inclusion of perspectives from colleagues who have worked across different countries and cultures, including Thailand, the UK, the Philippines, India, Ireland, and the Caribbean. Each chapter reflects not just a professional commitment to trauma-informed care but a genuine desire to share knowledge and practical approaches from diverse contexts, offering a global perspective on trauma and healing.

As editors and contributors, we have all worked in trauma care for many years, and this book represents not only our professional experiences but also our collective belief in the transformative power of trauma-informed care. It is our hope that by sharing our expertise, we can help others understand the profound impact of trauma and how we, as healthcare providers, can offer healing through compassion, understanding, and effective care.

I would like to extend my deepest gratitude to the colleagues who have contributed to this work. Your dedication to the care of trauma survivors and your willingness to share your expertise has made this book possible. Together, we have created a resource that will guide others in the critical work of trauma-informed care.

Baltimore, MD, USA   Tamar Rodney

Contents

1	**History of Trauma-Informed Care**	1
	Tamar Rodney	
2	**Post-traumatic Stress Disorder**	7
	Tamar Rodney	
3	**Community Trauma**	13
	Patty Wilson and Eugenia Millender	
4	**Trauma and Settings**	23
	Emma Mangano	
5	**Traumatic Physical Injuries and Mental Health Outcomes**	37
	Michelle Patch and Tamar Rodney	
6	**Trauma Experience and the Impact on Caregivers in Formal and Family Settings: Ethical Considerations**	47
	Georgina Morley and Louise Isham	
7	**Generational Trauma**	81
	Eugenia Millender and Patty Wilson	
8	**Cumulative Trauma**	93
	Michelle Patch and Tamar Rodney	
9	**Trauma Exposure and Symptom Presentations**	105
	Chitchanok Benjasirisan, Pearl Ed Cuevas, Veroina Deslandes, Rajesh Kumar, Tamar Rodney, Suratsawadee Kruahong, and Thitipong Tankampuan	
10	**Trauma Assessment**	125
	Tamar Rodney and Emma Mangano	
11	**Trauma: Biological Outcomes**	145
	Tamar Rodney	
12	**Trauma and Resilience**	151
	Tamar Rodney, Pearl Ed Cuevas, Thitipong Tankampuan, Rajesh Kumar, Veroina Deslandes, Chitchanok Benjasirisan, and Suratsawadee Kruahong	

13 Addressing Trauma: Behavioural Outcomes 165
   Tamar Rodney

14 Addressing Trauma: Reshaping the Future 171
   Chitchanok Benjasirisan, Pearl Ed Cuevas, Veroina Deslandes,
   Louise Isham, Suratsawadee Kruahong, Rajesh Kumar,
   Emma Mangano, Eugenia Millender, Georgina Morley,
   Michelle Patch, Tamar Rodney, Thitipong Tankampuan,
   and Patty Wilson

Contributors

Chitchanok Benjasirisan Johns Hopkins University School of Nursing, Baltimore, MD, USA

Pearl Ed Cuevas Centro Escolar University Manila, Manila, Philippines

Veroina Deslandes University of the West Indies-Mona, Kingston, Jamaica

Louise Isham Department of Social Work and Social Care, University of Birmingham, Birmingham, UK

Suratsawadee Kruahong Johns Hopkins University School of Nursing, Baltimore, MD, USA

Rajesh Kumar All India Institute of Medical Sciences, Rishikesh, Uttarakhand, India

Emma Mangano Johns Hopkins University School of Nursing, Baltimore, MD, USA

Eugenia Millender Florida State University, Tallahassee, FL, USA

Georgina Morley Center for Bioethics & Stanley S. Zielony Institute for Nursing Excellence, Cleveland Clinic, Cleveland, OH, USA

Michelle Patch Johns Hopkins University School of Nursing, Baltimore, MD, USA

Tamar Rodney Johns Hopkins University School of Nursing, Baltimore, MD, USA

Thitipong Tankampuan Mahidol University Faculty of Nursing, Bangkok, Thailand

Patty Wilson Johns Hopkins University School of Nursing, Baltimore, MD, USA

History of Trauma-Informed Care

Tamar Rodney

Objectives
- To describe the concept of trauma-informed care.
- To explore the inclusion in nursing assessment.
- To explore the inclusion in nursing treatment planning.
- Explore the inclusion of concepts in healthcare.

Introduction

Trauma Defined

Trauma has been described as "an emotional response to a terrible event like an accident, rape, or natural disaster" (Dalenberg et al. 2017). Not all stressful events involve trauma. The American Psychiatric Association's (APA) *Diagnostic and Statistical Manual of Mental Disorders* recommends that consideration of an event as a trauma requires "actual or threatened death, serious injury, or sexual violence" (APA 2022). When these event(s) are experienced as traumatic, the associated experiences can overwhelm an individual's capacity to cope, often resulting in feelings of helplessness, fear, and a loss of control. Traumatic events can be single incidents, such as accidents or assaults, or prolonged experiences, such as abuse or ongoing exposure to violence.

T. Rodney (✉)
Johns Hopkins University School of Nursing, Baltimore, MD, USA
e-mail: trodney1@jhu.edu

Trauma-Informed Care: The concept of trauma-informed care has evolved over the years as researchers and practitioners recognized the profound impact of trauma on individuals' well-being. The Substance Abuse and Mental Health Services Administration (SAMHSA) defines trauma-informed care as "a strengths-based service delivery approach that is grounded in an understanding of and responsiveness to the impact of trauma, that emphasizes physical, psychological, and emotional safety for both survivors to rebuild a sense of control and empowerment" (SAMHSA 2014). This approach has helped to support a paradigm shift in healthcare and other service sectors, aiming to create environments that prioritize safety, empowerment, and respect for individuals who have experienced trauma.

Inclusion in Nursing Assessment

For many nurses delivering a person-centred approach to care requires that a trauma-informed approach is maintained in all contexts of healthcare delivery and planning. This requires two main considerations:

1. Understand the role that violence and victimization play in the lives of individuals.
2. Apply that understanding to the design and delivery of service systems in order to accommodate the needs and vulnerabilities of trauma survivors and prevent retraumatization and or revictimization of those individuals.

A trauma-informed approach which is presented as the "Four Rs" by (SAMHSA) are Realize, Recognize, Responds, and Resists (see Fig. 1.1).

Recognition of Trauma History: Trauma-informed nursing assessment involves sensitively and proactively exploring patients' trauma histories. Healthcare providers inquire about traumatic experiences without triggering retraumatization and acknowledge the potential influence of trauma on the patient's current health status.

Trauma-Informed Approach (Four R's)

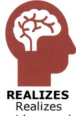

REALIZES Realizes widespread impact of trauma

RECOGNIZES Recognizes how trauma affects all individuals involved

RESPONDS Responds by putting this knowledge into practice

RESISTS Resists re-traumatization

Fig. 1.1 The Four Rs of trauma-informed care

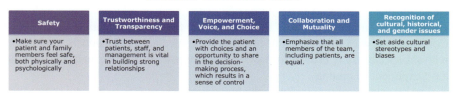

Fig. 1.2 Principles of trauma-informed care

Assessing Trauma-Related Symptoms: Nursing assessments include screening for trauma-related symptoms such as anxiety, depression, dissociation, and post-traumatic stress disorder (PTSD). Understanding the patient's trauma history helps tailor care plans to meet their unique needs. In addition, adherence to the five key principles of trauma-informed care allows nurses and healthcare professionals to recognize and respond with strategic guidance to the widespread impact that trauma can have on individuals and their families. These principles emphasize creating a safe and supportive environment while promoting healing and resilience (see Fig. 1.2).

Nurses have long been recognized as the most trusted profession, which increases the likelihood of individuals choosing to disclose information related to a history of trauma. In the nurse's role, there is a duty to act and responsibly provide sensitive care while prioritizing safety.

Knowledge of Trauma: Foundation for Action:
Understanding the nature of trauma is essential for effective care. This includes recognizing the varied manifestations of trauma, its effects on the brain and behaviour, and the potential long-term consequences.

Maintaining the safety of the environment and the individual involved is paramount in trauma-informed care. Individuals who have experienced trauma may have heightened sensitivity to perceived threats. Creating a physically and emotionally safe environment involves minimizing triggers, ensuring confidentiality, and establishing clear communication about boundaries and expectations. Safety also extends to the development of trust between nurse and individuals, emphasizing reliability and predictability in interactions.

Many of these disclosures may be historical in nature and include the experience of adverse childhood events (ACEs). Acknowledging the impact of ACEs is crucial in trauma-informed care. These events, such as abuse, neglect, or household dysfunction, can have lasting effects on mental and physical health. Mental health issues may include conditions like post-traumatic stress disorder (PTSD), anxiety, and depression. Physical health issues can arise due to the physiological impact of chronic stress. This may include increased risk of cardiovascular problems, immune system suppression, and other health concerns. Trauma-informed care addresses the interconnectedness of mental and physical health, recognizing that both aspects need attention and support. Trauma-informed care should also adopt a holistic approach that considers the whole person. This involves addressing not only the symptoms of trauma but also the underlying factors contributing to distress. Collaboration with mental health professionals, medical professionals, and other relevant specialists is crucial to provide comprehensive care for individuals who have experienced trauma.

The knowledge of trauma forms the foundation for creating a safe and supportive environment in care. Recognizing the prevalence of adverse childhood events and other traumatic experiences is vital, as is addressing the interconnectedness of mental and physical well-being. Adopting trauma-informed principles helps ensure that care is compassionate, empowering, and tailored to the unique needs of individuals who have experienced trauma.

Inclusion in Nursing Treatment Planning

Collaborative Approach: Trauma-informed nursing treatment planning involves a collaborative approach where the patient actively participates in the decision-making process. Providers respect the patient's autonomy and choices, recognizing that traumatic experiences may influence their responses to care.

Creating Safe Environments: Trauma-informed care emphasizes the importance of creating safe and supportive environments for patients. Nursing interventions focus on building trust, providing predictability, and ensuring physical and emotional safety during care delivery.

Inclusion of Concepts in Healthcare

Staff Training: Integrating trauma-informed care into healthcare requires training and education for all staff members. Healthcare providers receive education on trauma awareness, sensitivity, and understanding the impact of trauma on patient health.

System-Wide Changes: Trauma-informed care goes beyond individual interactions and extends to system-wide changes. Healthcare organizations adopt trauma-informed policies, procedures, and environmental modifications to support patients' healing and recovery.

Holistic Approach: Trauma-informed care recognizes that trauma affects multiple aspects of an individual's life. Therefore, healthcare providers address not only physical health but also mental, emotional, and social well-being in their care plans.

Summary

Trauma-informed care represents a critical shift in healthcare and other service sectors, recognizing the impact of trauma on individuals and guiding approaches that prioritize safety, empowerment, and compassion. Trauma-informed care should involve a recognition of the intersection of the prevalence of trauma and its potential contribution to various challenges, including mental health issues, substance abuse, and interpersonal difficulties. The inclusion of trauma-informed concepts in nursing assessment, treatment planning, and healthcare delivery contributes to patient-centred care that supports healing and recovery for those who have experienced trauma. As trauma-informed care continues to evolve, it remains a vital aspect of promoting resilience and well-being for all patients.

References

American Psychiatric Association (ed) (2022) Diagnostic and statistical manual of mental disorders, 5th edn. American Psychiatric Association, Arlington, VA

Dalenberg CJ, Straus E, Carlson EB (2017) Defining trauma. In: Gold SN (ed) APA handbook of trauma psychology: foundations in knowledge. American Psychological Association, pp 15–33

Substance Abuse and Mental Health Services Administration (2014) SAMHSA's concept of trauma and guidance for a trauma-informed approach. HHS Publication No. (SMA) 14-4884. Substance Abuse and Mental Health Services Administration, Rockville, MD

Post-traumatic Stress Disorder

2

Tamar Rodney

Objectives
- Describe trauma and stressor-related disorders.
- To explore the bio-psycho-social principles of post-traumatic stress disorder.
- To discuss the assessment of post-traumatic stress disorder.
- To describe current research related to post-traumatic stress disorder.

Introduction

Trauma and Stressor-Related Disorders

Trauma and stressor-related disorders are a group of mental health conditions that occur in response to traumatic experiences or significant stressors. These disorders are categorized by the Diagnostic and Statistical Manual of Mental Disorders as acute stress disorder, post-traumatic stress disorder (PTSD), adjustment disorders, disinhibited social engagement disorder, prolonged grief disorder, reactive attachment disorder, and other specified trauma- and stressor-related disorders (APA 2022).

Post-traumatic Stress Disorder (PTSD)

The American Psychiatric Association revised the classification of PTSD to be recognized as one of the trauma and stressor-related disorders in the 2013 publication of the DSM-5. This reflects a change from the previous classification as an

---

T. Rodney (✉)
Johns Hopkins University School of Nursing, Baltimore, MD, USA
e-mail: trodney1@jhu.edu

© The Author(s), under exclusive license to Springer Nature
Switzerland AG 2025
T. Rodney (ed.), *Trauma Informed Care*,
https://doi.org/10.1007/978-3-031-87526-7_2

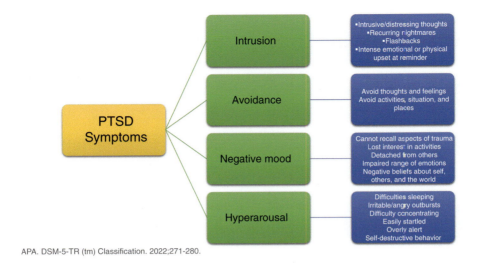

APA. DSM-5-TR (tm) Classification. 2022;271-280.

Fig. 2.1 PTSD symptom clusters

anxiety disorder. PTSD is a *psychiatric disorder that may develop in people who have a* history of trauma exposure involving actual or threatened death or serious injury to oneself or others (APA 2022). PTSD symptoms are organized into four symptom clusters (APA 2022) namely symptoms related to intrusion, avoidance, negative alterations in cognitions and mood, and alterations in arousal and reactivity as presented in the Diagnostic and Statistical Manual of Mental Disorders-5 (DSM-5-TR) (APA 2022). Each of these is described in Fig. 2.1. To receive a diagnosis of PTSD, individuals report at least one symptom from intrusive thoughts and avoidance clusters and at least two symptoms from negative thoughts and feelings and arousal and reactive symptoms clusters. Symptoms are experienced for more than a month, resulting in distress or functional impairment, and are not due to medication, substance use, or illness (Fig. 2.2). There are many publicly available screening tools for PTSD; however, the gold standard for diagnosing PTSD is a structured clinical interview such as the Clinician-Administered PTSD Scale (CAPS) (Weathers et al. 2017).

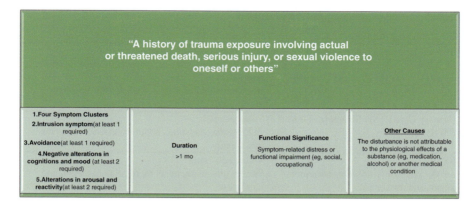

Fig. 2.2 PTSD diagnostic criteria (DSM-5-TR)

Bio-Psycho-Social Principles of Post-Traumatic Stress Disorder (PTSD)

Biological Factors: PTSD is associated with changes in brain functioning, particularly in regions related to fear, memory, and emotion regulation. Neurotransmitters, such as serotonin and norepinephrine, play a role in PTSD symptoms (Giotakos 2020; Sherin and Nemeroff 2011).

Psychological Factors: The experience of trauma can lead to the development of intrusive memories, nightmares, flashbacks, avoidance behaviours, and negative alterations in mood and cognition (van der Kolk 2000).

Social Factors: Social support and the quality of post-trauma social interactions influence the risk of developing PTSD. Strong support networks can mitigate the impact of trauma (Wang et al. 2021).

Trauma History Assessment

Nurses and all healthcare providers should approach trauma history assessment with sensitivity and empathy. Open-ended questions and non-judgemental language create a safe space for patients to share their experiences voluntarily. This can be done in the guided context of interviews or screening questions, utilizing

Table 2.1 Trauma screening and diagnosis tools

Screening and diagnosis tools	Considerations
Trauma Screening Questionnaire (TSQ)	10-item symptom screen Asks what they have experienced at least twice in the past week Recommended to give 3–4 week after traumatic event; cutoff: ≥6
Primary Care PTSD Screen for DSM-5 (PC-PTSD-5)	5-item screen Asks yes/no questions about experiences over the past month
SPAN startle, physically upset by reminders, anger, and numbness.	4-item self-report Startle, physically upset by reminders, anger, and numbness Assesses distress of items in the past week Item scored 0 (not at all distressing) to 5 (extremely distressing); score 5: positive
Short PTSD Rating Interview (SPRINT)	8-item self-report; 18+ year Assesses symptoms of PTSD in the past week Items scored 0 (not at all) to 4 (very much); cutoff: 14
PTSD Symptom Scale - Interview for DSM-5 (PSS-I-5)	24-item semi-structure interview Assesses symptoms of PTSD in the past month Items scored 0 (not at all) to 4 (6 or more times a week/severe)
Clinician-Administered PTSD Scale for DSM-5 (CAPS-5)	30-item structured interview Can be used to make a diagnosis, determine lifetime diagnosis Use by clinicians and clinical researchers with knowledge of PTSD

PTSD-related, age-appropriate screening tools. Nurses can utilize standardized screening tools, such as the PTSD Checklist for DSM-5 (PCL-5) or the Clinician-Administered PTSD Scale for DSM-5 (CAPS-5), to assess PTSD symptoms and severity. See Table 2.1.

Current Research Related to Post-traumatic Stress Disorder (PTSD)

Current research explores the neurobiological underpinnings of PTSD, focusing on the brain's response to trauma and the role of stress-related hormones. These discoveries include refining the process of identifying the cause of continued symptoms related to PTSD. These include the role of inflammation. There are several secondary injury cascades activated in response to trauma experiences, including inflammation (Sun et al. 2021). This response is mediated by a balance of inflammatory activities, which is orchestrated by cytokines (Rodney et al. 2018; Rodney et al. 2020). Exploring this relationship may lead to a greater understanding of the inflammatory responses to trauma and the development of PTSD.

Treatment Approaches

Research continues to investigate the effectiveness of various treatment modalities for PTSD. While there are two *selective serotonin reuptake inhibitors (SSRIs)*, with FDA approval for the treatment of PTSD symptoms available, there are no current pharmacotherapy options exclusive to PTSD. The first line of treatment remains the use of individual trauma-focused psychotherapy. These include cognitive-behavioural therapy (CBT), eye movement desensitization and reprocessing (EMDR), and complementary therapies (Table 2.2). A key component of treatment is the inclusion of utilizing a strengths-based approach including building resilience strategies. Research studies are ongoing to understand factors that contribute to resilience after trauma, as well as the development of preventive interventions to reduce the risk of PTSD in at-risk populations.

Table 2.2 Treatment of PTSD

Treatment option	Description
Cognitive processing therapy	Modify beliefs related to the trauma
	12 sessions; individual/structured group sessions
Cognitive behavioral therapy	Change thinking patterns
	Between 6 and 20 sessions; individual/group sessions
Cognitive therapy	Interrupt the behavioral and/or thought
	Weekly sessions over 3 month; individual/group sessions
Prolonged exposure therapy	Confront fears with imaginal and in vivo exposure
	8–15 sessions over 3 month; individual sessions
Eye movement desensitization and reprocessing	Lowering the intensity of negative thoughts and emotions
	8-phase treatment; individual sessions
Brief eclectic psychotherapy	Suppress intense emotions of sorrow
	16 sessions; individual sessions
Narrative exposure therapy	Imaginary trauma exposure, reorganizing memories
	4–12 sessions; individual sessions

Summary

Assessment, diagnosis, and treatment of PTSD are multidimensional processes that involve a comprehensive understanding of trauma and its effects on individuals. Clinicians approach trauma history assessment with sensitivity and employ standardized tools to assess PTSD symptoms and severity. PTSD treatment options continue to evolve, with ongoing research exploring the neurobiological basis of the disorder and the effectiveness of various therapeutic approaches. Continued research and understanding of PTSD will contribute to improved assessment, diagnosis, and treatment strategies, ultimately supporting individuals on their path to healing and recovery.

References

American Psychiatric Association (APA) (2022) Diagnostic and statistical manual of mental disorders (5th ed., text rev.; DSM-5-TR). American Psychiatric Publishing

Giotakos O (2020) Neurobiology of emotional trauma. Psychiatriki 31(2):162–171. https://doi.org/10.22365/jpsych.2020.312.162

Rodney T, Osier N, Gill J (2018) Pro- and anti-inflammatory biomarkers and traumatic brain injury outcomes: a review. Cytokine 110:248–256. https://doi.org/10.1016/j.cyto.2018.01.012

Rodney T, Taylor P, Dunbar K, Perrin N, Lai C, Roy M, Gill J (2020) High IL-6 in military personnel relates to multiple traumatic brain injuries and post-traumatic stress disorder. Behav Brain Res 392:112715. https://doi.org/10.1016/j.bbr.2020.112715

Sherin JE, Nemeroff CB (2011) Post-traumatic stress disorder: the neurobiological impact of psychological trauma. Dialogues Clin Neurosci 13(3):263–278. https://doi.org/10.31887/DCNS.2011.13.2/jsherin

Sun Y, Qu Y, Zhu J (2021) The relationship between inflammation and post-traumatic stress disorder. Front Psychiatry 12:707543. https://doi.org/10.3389/fpsyt.2021.707543

van der Kolk B (2000) Posttraumatic stress disorder and the nature of trauma. Dialogues Clin Neurosci 2(1):7–22. https://doi.org/10.31887/DCNS.2000.2.1/bvdkolk

Wang Y, Chung MC, Wang N, Yu X, Kenardy J (2021) Social support and posttraumatic stress disorder: a meta-analysis of longitudinal studies. Clin Psychol Rev 85:101998. https://doi.org/10.1016/j.cpr.2021.101998

Weathers FW, Bovin MJ, Lee DJ, Sloan DM, Schnurr PP, Kaloupek DG et al (2017) The clinician-administered PTSD scale for DSM-5 (CAPS-5): development and initial evaluation in military veterans. Psychol Assess 30(3):383–395

Community Trauma

Patty Wilson and Eugenia Millender

Objectives
- Describe the difference between individual-level trauma and community-level trauma
- Identify socio-cultural environmental, built environmental, and economic environmental symptoms of community trauma
- Identify adverse community experiences that can result in community trauma

Introduction

Traumatic experiences are not limited to individuals. Trauma can be collectively experienced, impacting entire groups of people, communities, or societies (Weisner 2020). Community trauma, also referred to as collective trauma, exists in the collective memory of individuals with shared experiences and social identity (Hirschberger 2018). The COVID-19 pandemic, political polarization, economic uncertainty, mass shootings, race-based violence, and natural disasters have led to a surge of collective traumas. Understanding that most often the approaches to address trauma are focused on individuals rather than communities, Pinderhughes et al. developed a framework for addressing community trauma (2015). The Prevention Institute's Adverse Community Experiences and Resilience Framework describes the experiences, conditions, and symptoms of trauma that adversely impact communities

P. Wilson (✉)
Johns Hopkins University School of Nursing, Baltimore, MD, USA
e-mail: pwilso23@jhu.edu

E. Millender
Florida State University, Tallahassee, FL, USA
e-mail: Emillender@fsu.edu

Table 3.1 Key definitions

Complex trauma	Exposure to multiple, often interrelated forms of traumatic experiences
Community trauma	Trauma that is experienced beyond the individual level. Trauma that impacts entire groups of people, communities, or societies. Often referred to as collective trauma
Social determinants of health	Conditions in the places where people live, learn, work, and play, which affect a wide range of health and quality of life risks and outcomes (CDC)
Structural inequities—types of discrimination	Historical, social, political and economic factors that shape disparities in society, including healthcare outcomes and access, housing, education, and other resources (Fiske et al.)
Social-cultural environments	Comprises personal and organizational relationships within a community. The context in which social and cultural factors influence health outcomes (IOM 2006)
Physical-built environments	The context in which physical/built environments influence health outcomes
Economic environments	The context in which economic factors influence health outcomes

(Pinderhughes et al. 2015). According to the framework, community-level symptoms of community trauma are identified in the social-cultural environment, the physical/built environment, and the economic environment and often include structural violence and marginalization (Pinderhughes et al. 2015). This chapter will discuss the impact of social-cultural, physical/built, and economic environments on community trauma and how structural inequities, discriminatory practices, and disasters can lead to community trauma. See key definitions in Table 3.1.

Individual and Community Trauma

The Substance Abuse Mental Health Service Administration (SAMHSA) defines trauma through the "three Es": (1) *Event* that is emotionally painful or distressing; (2) *Experienced* as abnormally intense or stressful; and (3) *Effects* physical and mental health which are adverse and lasting (2019). The pivotal study conducted by Felitti et al., revealed the negative impact of adverse childhood experiences (ACEs) on the health and well-being of individuals (1998). Felitti and his team determined exposure to ACE is linked to physical and mental health, and substance misuse in adults. The dose-response relationship between the number of ACEs an individual has experienced and their risk of health and social consequences, including maladaptive coping behaviours, such as alcohol misuse; chronic health conditions such as obesity, heart disease, and cancer; mental health conditions, such as depression and suicide attempts, adverse social conditions, and early mortality (Felitti et al. 1998). Considering the initial ACE study findings based on data from predominantly White, middle to upper-middle class individuals, an adapted version was developed for a more diverse population. An adapted version developed by the Philadelphia ACE study added five additional questions to gain insight on the impact of community-level adversities of a more socioeconomical and racially diverse population. The expanded Philadelphia ACE questionnaire's community-level indicators included witnessing violence, living in foster care, bullying, experiencing racism or discrimination, and feeling unsafe in your neighbourhood. Forty percent of Philadelphians had experienced four or more of these expanded community-level ACEs based on study findings (Pachter et al. 2017).

Complex Trauma

Beyond adverse childhood experiences, individuals may also suffer from chronic stressors. Chronic and complex traumas refer to ongoing or over a longer time such as community violence, structural violence, racism, discrimination, poverty, homelessness, domestic violence, and many other types of chronic and complex traumas (Allmark et al. 2014; Ferrer and Conley 2015). A trauma is considered acute if it impacts individuals and communities for a short time period, i.e., a national disaster such as a hurricane (Allmark et al. 2014).

Adverse Community Experiences

It is important to know that community trauma is most often rooted in social inequities such as racism, poverty, oppression, and erasure of culture/communities as seen in instances of forced assimilation (i.e. Native Americans; African Americans). In a literature review by King et al., various types of chronic/complex trauma in several different populations were included among the studies reviewed. Studies included oppressed or historically marginalized communities; Indigenous communities facing historical trauma; immigrant and refugee communities; rural communities; low-income communities; and communities experiencing community violence or race-based stress. Figure 3.1 provides a list of various adverse community experiences that are often associated with community-level trauma. Figure 3.2 provides an overview of the symptoms of community-level trauma, illustrating how adversity manifests across three interconnected areas: people, place, and equitable opportunities. People experience the effects of trauma through damaged social networks, increased tolerance for destructive social norms, and a diminished sense of collective efficacy. Place reflects trauma in the form of damaged public spaces and limited access to healthy products, contributing to an environment that reinforces stress and instability. Equitable opportunities are impacted as economic and educational disparities deepen, restricting access to resources that support long-term community resilience. The overlap of these three factors perpetuates cycles of trauma, making it essential to implement holistic, community-driven interventions that promote healing and stability.

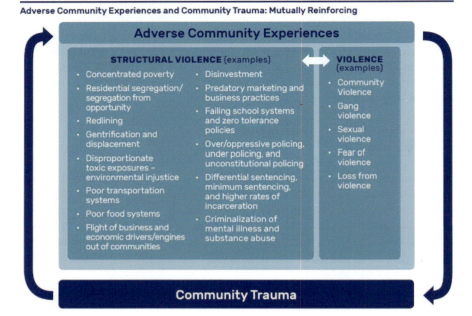

Fig. 3.1 Adverse community experiences

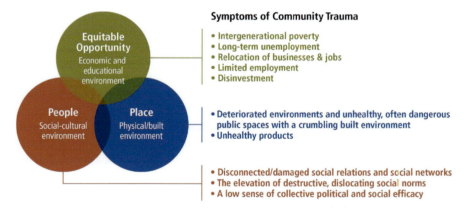

Fig. 3.2 Symptoms of community-level trauma

Potential Strategies to Reduce Community Trauma

The Adverse Community Experiences and Resilience Framework applies both prevention and intervention techniques to offer a holistic approach to addressing trauma. Table 3.2 lists strategies for communities to prevent and address trauma. According to Pinderhuges et al., "the most effective strategies build on Indigenous

Table 3.2 Potential strategies to reduce community trauma

Setting	Overall goal	Strategies	Potential applications
Physical	Safe spaces with cultural expression, quality housing, and availability of healthy products	Reclaiming, improving, and maintaining the physical space of the community	Maintaining the physical space of the communityPhysically improving outdoor spaces and buildings
		Creating safer public spaces	Increasing and maintaining parks, quality housing, and reliable public transportation
Social/cultural	Counter community trauma symptoms, support connection and healing, and establish norms that encourage healthy behaviours	Rebuild social relationships, social networks, and social support	Utilizing restorative justice within the community
		Promote social norms that encourage healthy behaviours	Implementing positive youth development programming
		Encourage collaboration and community-level solutions	Encourage relationships and communication between community organizations
		Provide community members a voice and restore/promote a sense of cultural identity	Organize regular, positive community activities
Economic/educational	Living wages, local wealth, and quality education	Support individuals to pursue educational and economic opportunities	Partner with local Big Brother, Big Sister programmes to provide mentoring and guidance to at-risk youth
		Develop strategies to improve the employment skills, capacity, and readiness of community members	Implement workforce development within the community
		Connect individuals with job opportunities, specifically those with a living wage	Work with workforce intermediaries that help to connect individuals with job opportunities
		Increase wealth and resources within communities	Promote economic opportunity, develop the workforce, and create a safe space for business relocation

Adapted from Pinderhughes et al. (2015)

knowledge, expertise, and leadership to produce strategies that are culturally relevant and appropriate (2015)". Understanding the factors that contribute to community trauma is essential for developing effective strategies to promote resilience and well-being. Figure 3.3 presents the Adverse Community Experiences and Resilience Framework. This framework identifies key factors within the social-cultural,

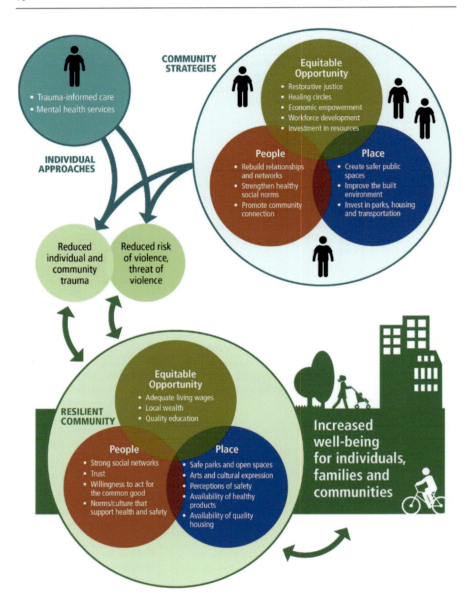

Fig. 3.3 Adverse Community Experiences and Resilience Framework. Adverse Community Experiences and Resilience Framework is drawn from Tool for Health and Resilience in Vulnerable Environments (THRIVE), a framework developed for the US Office of Minority Health by Prevention Institute to identify factors in the social-cultural, physical/built, and economic environments that contribute to health, safety, and well-being. (Source: Pinderhughes et al. 2015)

physical/built, and economic environments that influence community health, safety, and well-being. By examining how adverse experiences shape communities and exploring strategies for resilience, this framework provides a structured approach to addressing and preventing community trauma.

- Structural Inequities
  - Multiple types of discrimination—impacts the entire system
  - SDOH
    - Social-cultural environments
      - Concentrated poverty
      - Violence
      - Substance use
      - Social/recreational activities
      - Race-based trauma
    - Physical/built environments
      - Housing
      - Access to services: healthcare
      - Food deserts
      - Environmental hazards—lack of green space/lead/water
    - Economic environments
      - Education
      - Employment

The American Psychiatric Association (APA) defines trauma as an emotional response to an event, series of events, or circumstances that are perceived as harmful or life-threatening and have the potential to result in negative effects on an individual's physical, mental, and emotional or spiritual well-being (2013).

Case Studies

Case Study #1

A 19-year-old homeless Hispanic female, accompanied by her boyfriend, presents to a busy Emergency Department in downtown Los Angeles, California. At the hospital, she was diagnosed with advanced heart failure and her urine toxicology was positive for opiates, methamphetamine, and cannabis. Once her boyfriend leaves the room, she divulges that she was forced by her boyfriend to become a sex worker when she was 13 years old. She states "He got me addicted to drugs, now I shoot up [heroin] every day". Her mother and father, who immigrated from Mexico in their teens, have an extensive family history of mental illness, substance use, poverty, and housing instability. She states growing up she recalls her mother being admitted to the hospital often due to her longstanding paranoid schizophrenia. The patient had a child when she was 16 years old, which was an unintended pregnancy as a result of her "job". She was forced to put the child up for adoption by her boyfriend. She does not have a primary care provider, cardiologist, insurance, income, food that adheres to a cardiac diet, shelter, access to substance use treatment, or a consistent support system other than her boyfriend whom she shared is "the love of my life but also the devil".

1. What are examples of community trauma this patient has experienced?
2. How do you think the community-level trauma impacts this patient's health outcomes in the past, present, and future?

Case Study #2

Tia was a senior in college graduating in less than a month with only a few final exams left to take tomorrow. As she always does before exams, she went to her favourite restaurant near her college campus. As she was walking, she heard gunshots and immediately ran back to her apartment, locked the door, texted all of her college friends to see if they were safe, and turned on the news. The shooter was driving around an area of sororities and restaurants adjacent to campus, openly firing into the restaurants and targeting college girls like Tia. The news shared references to the shooter's YouTube channel and a 150-page manifesto which he shared with his therapist, family, teachers, and friends hours before the shooting describing his hatred of women, frustration about not being able to find a girlfriend, severe bullying he experienced as a child, contempt for interracial couples, and plan for retribution. The shooter was able to purchase two guns in the last several months from two nearby cities and plan his attack. He first stabbed 3 of his roommates to death before getting into his car and openly firing in the college campus adjacent community, ultimately killing 10 people and injuring 17 more. As Tia watched the news, she wondered how she, her friends, or any of the other students could ever possibly feel safe after this tragic massacre.

1. What types of emotional reactions may students like Tia and members of the surrounding community experience in the short term and long term after this traumatic event?
2. What prevention and/or intervention techniques would provide a holistic approach to addressing this community trauma and violence? Consider appropriate techniques at the individual, college community, city, county, state, and national levels.

Case Study #3

At the height of COVID-19 in Los Angeles, Mrs. Pruthi is devastated that she cannot host her yearly Diwali celebration, the most important religious festival in her

Indian community due to the mandatory "Stay-At-Home" order implemented by the county's mayor. Mrs. Pruthi misses and worries about her family in Punjab, India, getting sick and dying because COVID-19 cases are among the highest in the world, knowing that ten or more family members live in each of their five homes together and have no other places to quarantine safely or hospitals within a 50-mile radius. She is also reminded by her son, who is a doctor on the front lines treating COVID-19 in the hospital in Los Angeles, about the numerous deaths he sees daily and that there are no ICU beds available in Los Angeles during this devastating peak. Because Mrs. Pruthi is obese and sedentary with type II diabetes mellitus, hypertension, and hyperlipidemia, her son has been begging her to stay home because her medical conditions place her at a greater risk of developing severe illness if she were to get infected. Mrs. Pruthi has many friends like her with multiple comorbidities, several of whom have died or have loved ones who have died, and she thinks COVID-19 has impacted everyone's lives, some in more tragic ways than others. Mrs. Pruthi and her friends are often glued to the news channel on television and talk about how terrified they are that they will certainly die because of their vulnerability accompanied by inconsolable grief seeing the vast numbers of people dying in their own community and around the world. Mrs. Pruthi has been reassuring her son that she is staying at home most of the time now since her favourite volunteer activity that participating in with her LA Sikh community—handing out free food at the nearest temple, or Gurdwara, to anyone in need of food such as the homeless—has been shut down because of infectious potential. The homelessness crisis in Los Angeles existed prior to the pandemic, with 66,000 homeless persons in the county in 2020 and numbers continuing to rise as more and more employees are laid off from businesses, including restaurants, movie theatres, gyms, and retail stores, that have been temporarily or permanently shut down, and people can no longer afford high rates of rent. Mrs. Pruthi saw on the local news that the local government is working on an emergency shelter plan to slow the spread of COVID-19, but in the meantime, homeless shelters are shutting down when they inevitably experience outbreaks. Sad and discouraged, Mrs. Pruthi wonders how her communities of Los Angeles and Punjab ever recover if the pandemic ever comes to an end.

1. What types of individual-level trauma and community-level trauma can you distinguish in this narrative?
2. According to the Pinderhughes et al. (2015) framework, which strategies do you think should be prioritized to address community-level trauma associated with the COVID-19 pandemic aftermath?

Summary

This chapter delves into the intricate concept of community trauma, differentiating it from individual-level trauma. Collective trauma, also known as community trauma, affects entire groups, communities, or societies and is typically caused by social inequities such as racism, poverty, and oppression. We explore how sociocultural, physical/built, and economic environments can impact community trauma, including symptoms such as structural violence and marginalization.

To define trauma, we utilize the "three Es" framework, which highlights events that are emotionally distressing, experienced intensely, and have lasting adverse effects on physical and mental health. The impact of early trauma on health and well-being is demonstrated by adverse childhood experiences (ACEs) research. We also discuss chronic and complex traumas, such as community violence and discrimination, and acute traumas like natural disasters.

Furthermore, we highlight various adverse community experiences associated with community-level trauma, such as historical trauma in marginalized communities, immigrant and refugee experiences, and race-based stress. We present strategies to reduce community trauma, including creating safe physical spaces, rebuilding social relationships, promoting healthy behaviours, supporting education and economic opportunities, and fostering cultural identity.

Ultimately, this chapter offers valuable insights into the complexity of community trauma and suggests a framework for addressing and preventing it through culturally relevant and community-based strategies.

Discussion Questions

How does intersectionality impact community trauma with considerations for gender and ethnicity and sexual orientation?

References

Allmark P, Bhanbhro S, Chrisp T (2014) An argument against the focus on community resilience in public health. BMC Public Health 14:62. https://doi.org/10.1186/1471-2458-14-62

American Psychiatric Association (2013) Diagnostic and statistical manual of mental disorders, 5th edn. https://doi.org/10.1176/appi.books.9780890425596

Felitti VJ, Anda RF, Nordenberg D, Williamson DF, Spitz AM, Edwards V, Koss MP, Marks JS (1998) Relationship of childhood abuse and household dysfunction to many of the leading causes of death in adults. The Adverse Childhood Experiences (ACE) Study. Am J Prev Med 14(4):245–258. https://doi.org/10.1016/s0749-3797(98)00017-8

Ferrer B, Conley L (2015) Boston strong: the role of community resilience. J Public Health Manag Pract 21(Suppl 1):S34–S37. https://doi.org/10.1097/PHH.0000000000000133

Hirschberger G (2018) Collective trauma and the social construction of meaning. Front Psychol 9:1441. https://doi.org/10.3389/fpsyg.2018.01441

Institute of Medicine (2006) Improving the quality of health care for mental and substance-use conditions: Quality chasm series. The National Academies Press. https://doi.org/10.17226/11470

Pachter LM, Lieberman L, Bloom SL, Fein JA (2017) Developing a community-wide initiative to address childhood adversity and toxic stress: a case study of the Philadelphia ACE task force. Acad Pediatr 17(7):S130–S135

Pinderhughes H, Davis R, Williams M (2015) Adverse community experiences and resilience: a framework for addressing and preventing community trauma. Prevention Institute. Oakland CA

Weisner L (2020) Individual and community trauma: individual experiences in collective environments. Illinois Criminal Justice Information Authority

Trauma and Settings

Emma Mangano

Objectives
- Describe the various settings in which patients who have experienced trauma are often assessed
- Discuss creating a therapeutic setting for trauma victims across the lifespan
- Explain how to incorporate trauma-informed care into the emergency department, trauma centres and the primary care setting
- Compare how trauma is addressed in traditional versus non-traditional settings
- Describe how an interdisciplinary team addresses trauma in healthcare settings

Introduction

To discuss trauma, it is first important to understand how it is understood across disciplines. In psychiatric and mental health, trauma may indicate a history of violence or abuse. Within the emergency department, the announcement of an arriving trauma often indicates a serious physical injury, such as a gunshot wound. Furthermore, this definition can vary depending on the patient population. Trauma experienced by a veteran is vastly different from a young adult who has faced adverse childhood experiences (ACEs).

The Substance Abuse and Mental Health Services Administration (SAMHSA) in the United States notes that there are many definitions of trauma. This makes it difficult for a consensus on how to create a framework of care. After a review, SAMHSA (2014) provided clarity with the following concept:

E. Mangano (✉)
Johns Hopkins University School of Nursing, Baltimore, MD, USA
e-mail: ebarth3@jhmi.edu

Individual trauma results from an event, series of events, or set of circumstances that is experienced by an individual as physically or emotionally harmful or life threatening and that has lasting adverse effects on the individual's functioning and mental, physical, social, emotional, or spiritual well-being (p. 7).

When caring for a patient with a history of trauma, the nurse will have to reflect on this definition. SAMHSA refers to this as the "three E's" of trauma: events, experiences and effects (SAMHSA 2014). Is one person impacted or is an entire family impacted by one event? What lifespan considerations will need to be made and how will presentations differ based on developmental stages? How is the patient you are caring for defining the trauma?

People with a history of trauma may not always present initially in the mental health system. The experience of trauma and how one copes with the experience will not fit a textbook definition. The concept of trauma-informed approaches includes integrating knowledge about trauma into practice and policies and efforts to prevent re-traumatization of individuals and groups (Champine et al. 2019). This chapter will discuss the various settings in which nurses will encounter patients who have experienced trauma, how to provide trauma-informed care in these settings, and patient presentations that may suggest a history of trauma (Table 4.1). An overall theme the reader of this chapter is to remember—is not to ask, "what's wrong with you?" but rather "what happened to you?".

Table 4.1 Key elements of a trauma assessment across settings

Key element	Setting		
	High acuity	Ambulatory	Non-traditional
Screening	This will include asking patients during the triage and intake process. Chart reviews may need to be completed for patients unable to participate	Trauma screening tools (see Chap. 11) appropriate for the patient's developmental age. Nurses and providers can also screen as part of their routine exams	Prioritize care for medical needs. Assessment includes providing emotional support and screening for adverse reactions
Diagnosis	The nurse should be aware of common symptoms of a PTSD diagnosis that may be exacerbated in this setting. This includes the symptom cluster of changes in physical and emotional reactions. A definitive diagnosis is not likely to be made in this setting	In this setting, the nurse may find the patient presents with physical complaints that may be a complication of past trauma. A definitive diagnosis is not likely to be made in this setting; however, a positive screen may clue the PCP to a PTSD diagnosis	A diagnosis of acute stress disorder is most likely in this setting. The nurse may identify symptoms immediately following the event, but for diagnosis, must persist for 3 days and up to a month for a diagnosis

(continued)

4 Trauma and Settings

Table 4.1 (continued)

Key element	Setting		
	High acuity	Ambulatory	Non-traditional
Referral	An assessment of the level of distress or impairment will determine the appropriate next steps. Referrals in this setting may include an inpatient mental health admission, referral to a crisis bed or intensive outpatient programmes	A positive screen for PTSD or trauma should automatically trigger a referral to a mental health provider for an accurate diagnosis The nurse can also refer patients to resources in the community, such as support groups or therapists	Referrals in this setting are based on the person's most acute needs. This could be shelter, food security or mental health interventions. Government agencies may also be available and can be referred to for further support
Safety	In this setting, efforts should be made to create an environment of decreased stimulation and increased privacy. The patient should be included in care decisions to promote autonomy. Before invasive procedures, the patient should be made aware of what to expect and address questions or concerns. All efforts to avoid use of restraints and seclusion should be made by utilizing de-escalation techniques	Building rapport and a trusting relationship with the patient is the first step to creating a safe environment. Reinforcing privacy practices, except in cases of risk of harm to self or others, is also essential. Privacy should also be maintained if the patient is asked to remove clothing for exams. A review of what to expect during the visit should be made with an opportunity to address questions or concerns	Prioritization of basic needs (consider Maslow's Hierarchy of Needs) to create a safe environment. Allow for a space to have private conversations. Do not provide false reassurance, but rather a sense of hope

(continued)

Table 4.1 (continued)

Key element	Setting		
	High acuity	Ambulatory	Non-traditional
Follow-up	While a patient may not necessarily follow up in the true sense of the term in these settings, it is important to reinforce that emergency settings are open 24/7 for care. Develop a personalized safety plan that the patient can refer to in times of crisis. This author recommends the Stanley-Brown Safety Plan. Include a discussion of return precautions prior to final disposition. Discharge planning from the acute, inpatient setting should include the patient and those involved in their care outside the hospital. Follow-up can include mental health appointments, day programmes, plus a wide range of other services that may be available in the community. In both settings, the nurse should include the history of trauma during rounds and report to other nurses and providers	Utilization of electronic health records messaging systems provides a valuable opportunity to remain in close follow-up after a positive screen or referral. A phone call can be used if electronic messaging systems are not available. Communication and collaboration with outpatient mental health providers are essential to ensure the patient is meeting their goals towards recovery	In this setting, the nurse may remain a source of support for the person and help direct them to the necessary resources. Ensure a warm handoff to another nurse or point person if unable to return

High Acuity Settings

Emergency Department

The emergency department (ED), accident and emergency (A&E) area of a hospital, along with other acute care settings, such as an inpatient mental health unit, is the first area of discussion. This clinical setting can often be unpredictable in nature, and those providing care must be flexible with often changing scenarios. How a patient arrives can also vary and impact the care experience. Up to two-thirds of patients who present to an ED feel that they were coerced by law enforcement or other prehospital staff and subsequently led to an agitated arrival experience (Wong et al. 2020). This can then have an impact on the ability to forge a therapeutic relationship. Agitation and interventions by healthcare staff can also be traumatizing or re-traumatizing for acutely ill patients.

Trauma-informed care can be difficult to provide in high-volume and high-acuity environments (Jordan 2019). This is true of most clinics or units that have an unpredictable setting. Traumatic memories or fears can be triggered by overstimulation or loud noises (Molloy et al. 2020). To begin providing care for a patient, whether for physical or psychiatric emergencies, a therapeutic environment should be created. The first step is to create a welcoming, non-threatening environment that promotes a sense of safety and security (Jordan 2019). Inform the patient of the next steps in the evaluation and what to expect. This creates a culture of trust. Simple medical procedures, such as the tightening of a blood pressure cuff, can be reminiscent of being held against one's will. For procedures that can be painful, pre-medication should be given and a source of distraction considered. If possible, a supportive caregiver should also be present (Jordan 2019).

Acute Mental Health

In other settings, such as inpatient mental health or crisis units, these same principles apply. Patients with a history of trauma are more often to leave against medical advice (AMA) if the environment of the milieu is chaotic or interpreted to be unsafe. Some reasons for this may be due to the decreased autonomy of such units, the hierarchal structure of an organization, the unfamiliar surroundings, or the presence of other agitated or aggressive patients (Gatov et al. 2020). Witnessing or being part of restraint and seclusion events can also be re-traumatizing for patients. Both interventions are considered failures of care, as they are used when all previous interventions for patient safety have not been effective. The use of force, including short-term holds, holds for medication, physical escort and the placing of restraints, is often viewed as traumatic. They can lead to flashbacks or be re-traumatizing. For example, if a woman has been a victim of rape, the use of force and restraint can cause more harm than the purpose of this safety intervention. In this scenario, it is important to prioritize the use of female nursing and security staff.

The likelihood that a nurse will care for a patient that has a trauma history is high; it has been found that 46–89% of those who use mental health services have been exposed to previous trauma (Molloy et al. 2020). On inpatient psychiatric units, 40% of women and 25% of men have a history of interpersonal trauma (Gatov et al. 2020). The nurse is often the one responsible for delivering trauma-informed care and leading the interdisciplinary team in preventing re-traumatization.

Special Populations

Although paediatric presentations represent a small proportion of all ED visits at 20 percent, many will present for physical assault-related injuries. It is believed there are over 1000 visits per day for such concerns (McDermott et al. 2006; SAMHSA 2023). In the initial assessment of the paediatric patient, it is recommended that the nurse remembers that the behaviour and health status of the patient could be impacted by previous trauma. Thus, it is important to be asking "what happened" to the child rather than "what's wrong" with them. Statements should also not provide false reassurance, which could lead to stress or discomfort (Jordan 2019). The acute setting can be frightening or unfamiliar to a child. The nurse can create a trusting and therapeutic environment by providing clear statements about what is happening and allowing them to make decisions in their care (Jordan 2019).

Patients with cognitive deficits, similar to paediatric patients, may also have difficulty expressing what they have experienced. Their vulnerability continues to put them at increased risk for abuse as they may not be able to communicate events that are ongoing or may not be aware that they are being abused or taken advantage of (Dorney-Smith et al. 2020). Another group that is more likely to have been exposed to ACEs and trauma are those experiencing homelessness. This population can present with post-traumatic stress disorder (PTSD) or personality traits that can lead to challenges and disruption in care. The nurse may find that this patient population has difficulty trusting others, managing stress or waiting for treatment. To prevent disruptive behaviours, which could lead to violence and removal from the setting, the nurse should use calm and professional language (Dorney-Smith et al. 2020). This allows the patient an opportunity to tell the nurse what the situation is, in a safe and welcoming environment.

The Interdisciplinary Team

As previously mentioned, the nurse in the acute care setting will need to plan their approach to care and will have the responsibility of coordinating with the interdisciplinary team to prevent re-traumatization. This process begins in triage. The assessment should include a thorough medical history that includes both mental health and substance use history (Dorney-Smith et al. 2020). Creating this open and nonjudgmental dialogue allows for the patient to be viewed as a whole person, not just the "chief complaint". The next step in the process is completing role induction. This process, which often involves the interdisciplinary team but is initiated by the nurse, ideally begins when a patient is brought onto a new unit. During role induction, the patient is made aware of the unit policies, expectations of their care, and the relationships and roles of each team member. This also includes patient expectations. It is also important to keep the expectations realistic. Although particularly important for the paediatric patient, this final concept is generalizable across all populations. In acute care settings, the nurse often has multiple responsibilities, including caring for individuals with a variety of needs. Regardless, the nurse must continue to maintain a safe and trustworthy environment. This can include introducing new team members or when procedures are necessary. By showing that they care, specifically with the paediatric patients, it can have a lasting impact on outcomes (Jordan 2019).

There can also be times when a patient's background is unknown, and behaviours displayed may be indicative of past trauma. In this situation, the team should make every attempt to obtain collateral information to prevent further harm and trauma. As a team, open communication and updates should be continuously flowing. Changes happen often and frequently in this setting, including the patient's status. For example, disruptive behaviours can be indicative of maladaptive coping in response to a patient's history. In this situation, the team should prioritize understanding what the patient has experienced for this to occur, provide clear information about the situation, display trust and offer solutions (Dorney-Smith et al. 2020). Within inpatient mental health units, there will also be a group of patients with a history of past trauma but not necessarily meet diagnostic criteria for PTSD. It has been found that for patients with primary substance use diagnoses that had undesirable outcomes on disposition, trauma was minimally reported (Gatov et al. 2020). Regardless of a PTSD diagnosis, the team must continue to set a trusting environment and optimal outcomes. "Best practice through a trauma-informed approach can be attained only when all team members contribute their unique specialized knowledge and skill set in a collaborative effort to achieve the common goal of [child] safety and protection" (Jordan 2019, p. 319).

Ambulatory Care Settings

The ambulatory care setting or primary care setting is another unique space where nurses may encounter caring for patients with a history of trauma. The role of the nurse in these settings is different than previously discussed. These appointments are expected and predictable. A significant portion of the visit is spent with the primary care provider (PCP), making the role of the nurse critical. The utilization of screening and diagnostic tools is critical to communicate current well-being and baseline health with providers. The appropriate next steps in care, including referrals, should be guided by the nurse.

One of the first indications that a patient may be a victim of trauma may be from the physical symptoms they present with and not necessarily those that are psychiatric in nature. Patients can present with neurologic sequelae from head traumas, chronic health conditions like diabetes or heart disease, prolonged inflammatory response, decreased healing and insulin resistance (Palmieri and Valentine 2021). For this reason, the recommendation is to assume that your patient has experienced trauma at some point in their lifetime and care approaches should be directed with this in mind (Palmieri and Valentine 2021). In fact, patients who were recently discharged from an inpatient mental health unit with a history of trauma were more likely to follow up with their PCP in the next 30 days than a psychiatrist (Gatov et al. 2020).

A benefit of this setting for trauma assessments is the predictability and safety of that environment. Often, the PCP has developed a relationship with the patient over time and there is mutual trust. This relationship is important in understanding that a patient's presentation or concerns and physical health may be a result of events that were, or currently are, out of their control (Roberts et al. 2019). To build on this trust, remind the patient that everything remains confidential unless they or someone else is in immediate danger. This could include having to disclose a duty to warn or involving emergency services if there is a risk of suicide.

A model for incorporating trauma-informed care into primary care (TIPC) is based on the key elements of trauma informed care (TIC): recognition, realization, response, respect and resilience (Roberts et al. 2019). In TIPC, the first component is screening and trauma recognition. The model continues with understanding the health effects of trauma, patient-centred communication and care, emphasizing emotional safety and avoiding triggers, and knowledge of helpful treatment for trauma patients. Table 4.1 provides suggestions for how to approach the various aspects of trauma-informed care in each of the settings discussed.

Once a therapeutic environment is established, the assessment can begin. Again, it is important to emphasize the need to ask about trauma in a way that normalizes the question and ensuing discussion (Palmieri and Valentine 2021), similar to how a nurse would ask when a patient's last bowel movement occurred. The nurse should utilize open and non-threatening body language and provide anticipatory guidance about the visit. This includes non-invasive procedures, like obtaining vital signs, to those that could be re-traumatizing, such as a breast exam (Fleishman et al. 2019). The nurse in this situation can set the scene for a successful visit. Having a consistent team that is well-known to patients across the lifespan will provide the trust required if a referral to a mental health provider is needed (Balch and Loomis 2017). The ability to provide referrals is key to preventing misdiagnoses, particularly in the paediatric population where their behaviours are often attributed to attention deficit and hyperactivity disorder (ADHD) (Balch and Loomis 2017).

During the screening process, the nurse will work closely with other team members to ensure the best outcomes for the patient. Because patients are more often to see the PCP, than a mental health provider, a collaborative care model can be utilized to mitigate anxiety, reduce the need for acute care use, and unhealthy behaviours such as self-harm (Balch and Loomis 2017; Gatov et al. 2020). The team can also educate the patient about the connection between physical health and trauma. However, it is just as important to be able to make a referral to a trauma expert or mental health provider and community resources, such as support groups. The patient should also be allowed to decline a referral, with the team supporting this decision and reinforcing the benefits of specialized care at each interaction.

Reporting Suspected Abuse or Neglect

Nurses in both ambulatory and high-acuity settings may find that they are the first to learn about neglect or abuse. Within the United States, anyone may file a report if they suspect the welfare or safety of someone is in jeopardy. However, within each State, there are differences in who is mandated to report suspected abuse. In general, most professionals who work with children or vulnerable adults are mandated by law to report their concerns to child and adult protective services. For example, in the state of Maryland, health practitioners, educators or human service workers and police officers are professionals who are required to report known and suspected child abuse or neglect. Mandated reporters of suspected abuse or neglect of a vulnerable adult in Maryland include health practitioners, police officers, human service workers, and, in the case of financial exploitation, any banking institution (MD-DHS 2023).

Currently, in England, there is not a legal requirement for those who work with children to report known or suspected abuse. There is statutory guidance that recommends anyone who is concerned about a child's welfare make a referral to the appropriate authorities. This guidance is not a legal requirement, but it does require practitioners and organizations to take it into account and provide clear reasons why they did not if they did not comply. While concern about this has been brought to the government's attention, it was decided that there were several risks associated with a duty to act (Foster 2025).

Mandatory reporting laws are noted in other countries, including Australia, Brazil, Canada, Denmark, France, Hungary, the Republic of Ireland, Israel and Norway. Variation exists within each country, but the laws include who is covered by the duty, what must be reported, who the report must be made to, and sanctions for failing to report (Foster 2025). It is also important to note that what is considered a minor, or child, and adult can vary within and across countries (Box 4.1).

Box 4.1: Legal Definitions of Age Groups Within the United States

Minor: persons under the age of 18 years. They must be under the care of a parent or guardian.

Emancipated Minor: an eligible minor that is granted some or all rights and statuses of an adult. Must go through the process of emancipation, which is based on individual state laws. These laws specify when and the conditions that must be met for a child to become independent of their parents for legal purposes.

Adult: considered the "age of majority" and comes with the rights and responsibilities of adulthood. Many countries have this age set at 18 years; however, within the United States, it varies, with 19 years the age of majority in Nebraska and Alabama and 21 years in Mississippi.

Vulnerable Adult: those over the age of 18 years who do not have the physical or mental capacity to provide for their daily needs. Not necessarily a senior citizen. Includes those with cognitive limitations or developmental delays.

Incapacitated Adult: an adult that lacks the physical or mental ability to manage their own personal care, property or finances. This adult is not able to understand or communicate responsible decisions.

Guardian: appointed by the court to care for a person who is not able to take care of themselves. They are to protect the person, often referred to as the "ward". Guardians are regulated by state and local statutes and are monitored by the courts after appointment given their level of control over the wards' life and assets. Must act in their wards' best interest.

From Cornell Law School: Legal Information Institute

Vulnerable adult from Maryland Attorney General: https://www.marylandattorneygeneral.gov/MFCU%20Documents/VulnerableAdult.pdf

Community and Non-traditional Settings

Non-traditional settings in which the nurse may encounter those who have experienced trauma include schools and community settings following a disaster. In response to disasters, the focus will be on the ability to triage and assess those at high risk for an acute stress reaction or maladaptive coping mechanisms. With minimal response to address climate change, there will continue to be an increase in natural disasters, including stronger hurricanes and fires. The year 2020 was also a reminder of the impact a global pandemic can have on the health and well-being of local communities. The list only continues to grow as the world continues to face challenges from mass casualty events to displacement from internal conflicts.

Schools

The school nurse works in a non-traditional, ambulatory setting where many students have the opportunity to interact with the healthcare system. School, for most students, is a safe and supportive environment. Students may disclose information about their home life, including exposure to trauma, and the nurse will need to know how to respond appropriately. Unfortunately, best practice guidelines in this setting are not yet well established. The few studies that have been completed for school-based screening procedures and identifying youth exposed to trauma support a best practice (Eklund and Rossen 2016). Further complicating the situation is that parental permission may need to be obtained to do screening. If there is a positive screen, the school must be able to do the appropriate referral, while maintaining trust with both the child and family involved.

To address this lack of best practice, Eklund and Rossen (2016) discuss the "trauma-informed school". In this approach, schools understand that students with disruptive or problematic behaviour are reflective of a coping mechanism. School nurses and staff move away from asking what is wrong with the student, but rather what happened to the student. These behaviours are developed in response to their life experiences. A trauma-informed school should include the following (Eklund and Rossen 2016):

1. A school-wide focus, with policies and practices directed at all students, rather than only those impacted by trauma
2. A safe school environment
3. Building student capacities by teaching skills to learn resilience and coping
4. Building staff capacities through professional development and educational strategies to support students who have experienced trauma

Community Settings

The role of the nurse in these settings will also be non-traditional. Settings could include the local YMCA or an event stadium. Following a disaster or other incident, the nurse may find themselves as a care provider for a victim and not in the traditional nursing role. While the most important thing to do immediately after such an event is to address medical and life-threatening injuries, addressing emotional health will be just as important. Research shows that there is a link between exposure to trauma and healthcare needs immediately following the event and years later. This includes cardiovascular, neurological and psychiatric diagnoses (Sumner et al. 2023). Providing emotional support following a disaster can have a positive impact on the person cared for, even if the immediate effects are not seen.

Creating a therapeutic environment will not be an easy task. However, we again reiterate the need for safety and trust. A simple introduction can go a long way and create the opportunity for dialogue. Understand what the person's immediate needs are by considering Maslow's Hierarchy of Needs. Is there a need for food or water, warmth and clothing, or shelter? Addressing these simple, yet important needs will also lead to a safe environment. The nurse should consider them part of the therapeutic environment as well, especially when the physical environment may be in chaos or disarray. To do this, the nurse should remain calm and present, keeping focus on the person in distress. After a disaster and traumatic event, the person may find that they are unable to describe effectively what they have experienced. The nurse will need to help the person process their emotions, be an active listener and validate their feelings. Once safety has been secured, the nurse will have the responsibility of knowing the resources available and referring the person appropriately.

Case

Ms K is a 39-year-old Caucasian woman that has walked into a busy, urban emergency department requesting help with substance use. She is quickly registered but has been requested to remain in the waiting room until the triage nurse is available. While waiting, she decides to go outside to smoke a cigarette and upon returning, she learns that she missed her call from the triage nurse. She approaches the nursing area but is stopped by the male security guard. He attempts to redirect her by gently taking her arm to go back to the waiting area. This leads to her quickly escalating, yelling expletives towards the guard. The triage nurse, who is also a man, approaches the two to help de-escalate the situation. Ms K sees him approaching and escalates further and attempts to run away, resulting in a Code Green (for a violent patient) to be called overhead.

You are the nurse working in the psychiatric area of the ED today and were made aware of the patient when she initially registered. With the resulting Code Green, it is most likely that she will be escorted to psychiatry.

1. What are your initial steps in preparing to take care of Ms K prior to her arrival?
2. How will you prevent further escalation when Ms K comes into your care?

Unfortunately, on arrival, the covering physician orders her to receive intramuscular medications to "sedate" her. Ms K states she does not need the medication and that she will calm down on her own; however, the physician feels it is in her best interest. Shortly after receiving the medication, Ms K falls asleep in her room. As the nurse, you decide to review her chart to better understand Ms K and what led her to become violent.

3. What parts of Ms K's history will be pertinent to know for your ongoing care of her?
4. How can you support Ms K when she wakes up so that she can feel safe and supported?

When Ms K wakes up, she apologizes for what happened on her arrival and requests to speak with you as her nurse. She confides that when she was younger, a male security guard at her high school who looked similar to the hospital's guard, sexually assaulted her. She dealt with this on her own for most of her adult life, as her father was incarcerated for her childhood, and her mother did not believe her. "She told me I was just trying to get attention from the school". As a result, to cope with her trauma symptoms (anxiety, difficulty sleeping), she started to drink alcohol which was initially helpful. Soon, she found she had to drink almost all day, every day to keep herself from going into withdrawal. She has been unsuccessful in her attempts at sobriety and recovery.

5. How does Ms K's history explain her reactions when she initially presented to the ED? How do you develop rapport with Ms K so that you can deliver the best care?
6. After talking with Ms K and developing a rapport with her, she discussed with you that her goal is to get into a recovery programme. What resources in the community should be utilized to ensure her success and continue feeling supported?

Summary

Nurses make up the largest, single profession in the healthcare field. The jobs and responsibilities vary from the bedside to the school system to the boardroom. Wherever encountered, the nurse is most likely to be one of the first people the patient is to meet in the health system. In this chapter, three broad categories of settings were discussed where a nurse is likely to care for a patient with a history of trauma. High-acuity settings, such as the emergency department, are never areas that patients plan to visit. The unpredictable nature and highly stimulating environment can be a traumatizing experience for many patients. Nurses here should focus on understanding the patient's history and prevent re-traumatization. In the ambulatory setting, nurses should reinforce the importance of screening all patients for a history of trauma. This can help identify patients who may need resources beyond the primary care clinic. In non-traditional settings, the goal for the nurse is to meet the patient where they are following a potentially traumatic event.

4 Trauma and Settings

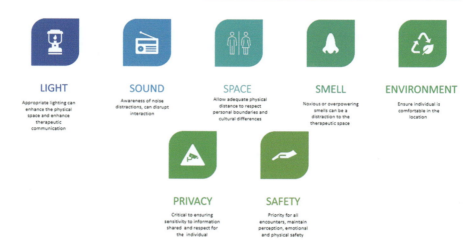

Fig. 4.1 Creating a therapeutic setting

Regardless of where the encounter is, the nurse should recognize and respond to the patient's history so that the best patient outcomes can occur (Palmieri and Valentine 2021). Creating a therapeutic environment that allows the patient to feel safe to discuss their history is also important (Fig. 4.1). In these settings, the nurse can further use themselves as a therapeutic tool and allow the patient to feel vulnerable. This, in turn, will provide the opportunity for the patient and nurse to build a trusting relationship in both the short and long term.

Discussion Question

Globally, many of the above settings will not be able to provide a space specifically designed for those who are in distress and benefit from a private setting, like Ms K. Think about your current practice location or where you have received care in the past. Is this setting prepared to care for those who have experienced trauma? As a nurse, what can you do to ensure your practice site is committed to care for trauma victims? What are the negative impacts of care if a patient does not feel safe or does not have privacy?

Concepts

Acute
Ambulatory/walk-In
Community setting
Emergency department
Trauma centres
Primary care setting

Interpersonal trauma
Therapeutic environment
Trauma-informed care

References

Balch MS, Loomis J (2017) Enhancing care models to capture psychological trauma. J Psychosoc Nurs Ment Health Serv 55(4):29–36

Champine RB, Lang JM, Nelson AM, Hanson RF, Tebes JK (2019) Systems measures of a trauma-informed approach: a systematic review. Am J Community Psychol. 64(3-4):418–437. https://doi.org/10.1002/ajcp.12388

Dorney-Smith S, Schneller K, Swift A, Phelan H, Khan Z (2020) Meeting the needs of homeless people attending the emergency department. Emerg Nurse 28(4):31–39

Eklund K, Rossen E (2016) Guidance for trauma screening in schools: a product of the defending childhood state policy initiative. The National Center for Mental Health and Juvenile Justice, Delmar

Fleishman J, Kamsky H, Sundborg S (2019) Trauma-informed nursing practice. Online J Issues Nurs 24(2). https://doi.org/10.3912/OJIN.Vol24No02Man03

Foster D (2025) Duties to report child abuse in England (Research Briefing). House of Commons Library. https://researchbriefings.files.parliament.uk/documents/SN06793/SN06793.pdf

Gatov E, Koziel N, Kurdyak P, Saunders NR, Chiu M, Lebenbaum M et al (2020) Discharge and post-discharge outcomes of psychiatric inpatients with a lifetime history of exposure to interpersonal trauma: a population-based study. Gen Hosp Psychiatry 65:82–90

Jordan KS (2019) Minimizing pediatric traumatic stress through a trauma-informed approach in the emergency department. J Emerg Nurs 45(3):319–322

Maryland Department of Human Services, Office of Adult Services (2023) Adult Protective Services – Investigating financial exploitation and abuse and access to records (Policy No. N/A). U.S. Department of Health and Human Services. https://dhs.maryland.gov/

McDermott KW, Stocks C, Freeman WJ (2006) Overview of pediatric emergency department visits, 2015. In: Healthcare cost and utilization project (HCUP) statistical briefs. Agency for Healthcare Research and Quality (US)

Molloy L, Fields L, Trostian B, Kinghorn G (2020) Trauma-informed care for people presenting to the emergency department with mental health issues. Emergency nurse: the journal of the RCN Accident and Emergency Nursing Association. 28(2):30–35. https://doi org/10.7748/en.2020.e1990

Palmieri J, Valentine JL (2021) Using trauma-informed care to address sexual assault and intimate partner violence in primary care. J Nurse Pract 17(1):44–48

Roberts SJ, Chandler GE, Kalmakis K (2019) A model for trauma-informed primary care. J Am Assoc Nurse Pract 31(2):139–144

Substance Abuse and Mental Health Services Administration (2014) SAMHSA's Concept of Trauma and Guidance for a Trauma-Informed Approach (HHS Publication No. (SMA) 14-4884). Substance Abuse and Mental Health Services Administration

Substance Abuse and Mental Health Services Administration (2023) Fiscal Year 2024: Justification of estimates for appropriations committees. U.S. Department of Health and Human Services. https://www.samhsa.gov/sites/default/files/samhsa-fy-2024-cj.pdf

Sumner JA, Cleveland S, Chen T, Gradus JL (2023) Psychological and biological mechanisms linking trauma with cardiovascular disease risk. Transl Psychiatry. 13(1):25. https://doi.org/10.1038/s41398-023-02330-8

Wong AH, Ray JM, Rosenberg A, Crispino L, Parker J, McVaney C, Iennaco JD, Bernstein SL, Pavlo AJ (2020) Experiences of individuals who were physically restrained in the emergency department. JAMA Netw Open. 3(1):e1919381. https://doi.org/10.1001/jamanetworkopen.2019.19381

Traumatic Physical Injuries and Mental Health Outcomes

5

Michelle Patch and Tamar Rodney

Objectives
- Discuss possible sources of traumatic physical injuries
- Briefly review the concept of inflammation
- Describe three nursing theories that address mind-body connectedness
- Explore various psychological responses to physical trauma
- Describe holistic nursing interventions for patients and families after physical trauma

Introduction

Traumatic physical injuries can come from many sources, whether natural (e.g. hurricanes, tornadoes, pandemics) or human-made (e.g. terrorist activity) and can be accidental (e.g. falls) or intentional (e.g. interpersonal violence) (Herrera-Escobar et al. 2021). How an individual categorizes the cause of physical injury influences their experience of trauma (e.g. locus of control, depersonalization) (APA 2022). The unexpected nature of an injury may lead to shock and fear for the individual, their family and loved ones, and the greater community. Physical injuries can trigger memories and re-living of the traumatic experience, uncovering unexplored vulnerabilities that may indicate the need for specialized referrals (SAMHSA 2014).

Further complexity and variability in presentation may be influenced by age, sex and gender identity, social economic status, life experiences, and other social and environmental determinants. For example, survivors of certain types of traumas, such as rape, may not consistently receive the same level of social empathy as other

M. Patch (✉) · T. Rodney
Johns Hopkins University School of Nursing, Baltimore, MD, USA
e-mail: mpatch1@jhmi.edu; trodney1@jhu.edu

© The Author(s), under exclusive license to Springer Nature Switzerland AG 2025
T. Rodney (ed.), *Trauma Informed Care*,
https://doi.org/10.1007/978-3-031-87526-7_5

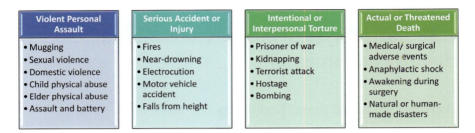

Fig. 5.1 Examples of physically traumatic events DSM-5TR

types of trauma survivors, like those involved in an accidental motor vehicle crash (Krug et al. 2002). Societal empathy for the cause of the trauma can significantly influence help-seeking and/or resource allocation. Adverse events in medical settings, although inadvertent, can result in survivor mistrust and reluctance to seek additional care, further distancing them from both physical and psychological support options. Physical injuries like burns, fractures, or amputation can require lengthy healing and therapy, with associated pain, frustration, and stress (Balikji et al. 2022). Traumatic or anoxic brain injuries can also cause cognitive impairment, mood alterations, and impulse control challenges (Robert 2020). Consideration of the source of trauma is a critical component in the nursing assessment and planning of care (see Fig. 5.1 for examples of physically traumatic events).

Caring for the health and well-being of trauma survivors requires we consider this interplay of physical and psychological injuries. Examining inflammation's role in mental health presentations after physical injury helps explain how it may further contribute to symptoms, morbidity, and mortality risks. It also offers insight into mental health assessment approaches, patient education, and treatment planning to mitigate these health risks.

Application of Trauma-Related Concepts and Research

Inflammation

After physical injury, our cells activate several pathways to provide protection and initiate healing (Fig. 5.2). These inflammatory activities have specific roles in recovery but can lead to excessive cellular damage as well as long-term structural and functional deficits if prolonged (Hori and Kim 2019; Rodney et al. 2018).

From: Rodney et al. (2018)

Hypothalamic–Pituitary–Adrenal (HPA) Axis

An acute stressor will trigger the sympathetic nervous system to secrete epinephrine and norepinephrine to help the body quickly respond to the threat. Increases in these hormones trigger the hypothalamus to release corticotropin-releasing hormone,

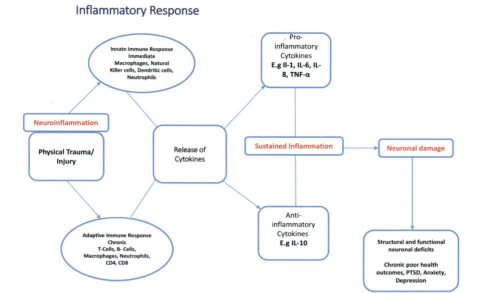

Fig. 5.2 Inflammatory pathway after injury

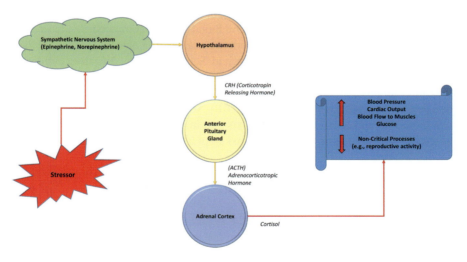

Fig. 5.3 Hypothalamic–pituitary–adrenal axis

leading then to the release of adrenocorticotropic hormone from the anterior pituitary gland. ACTH signals the adrenal cortex to release cortisol, leading to increased blood pressure, cardiac output, and glucose, helping skeletal muscles to react. Cortisol also decreases non-critical processes, such as reproductive activity, to allow the body to focus on the threat at hand (see Fig. 5.3, informed by Chrousos 2009). However, prolonged or chronic cortisol release has been associated with cardiovascular disease, immune system dysfunction, diabetes, obesity, memory and cognitive dysfunction, and mood disorders.

Epigenetic Changes

The heritability of adverse childhood experience (ACE) related phenotypes such as PTSD, depression, and resilience is low to moderate, and, moreover, is variable for a given phenotype, which implies that gene by environment interactions (such as through epigenetic modifications) may be involved in the onset of these phenotypes (Jiang et al. 2019). Research reporting epigenetic changes is still nascent, with preliminary evidence from both human and animal models (Jiang et al. 2019; Thumfart et al. 2022), and further research is warranted.

Depression, Anxiety, Trauma-Related Disorders (PTSD)

Research on mood disorders has demonstrated an interaction between genes and the environment among those with genetic predisposition, epigenetic regulation, and environmental effects (Breton et al. 2021). Along with multiple environmental factors, the experience of childhood trauma can relate to the pathogenesis, course, and treatment of mood disorders (Quidé et al. 2020). Individuals with mood disorders have reported a greater frequency of childhood trauma compared to the general population, and adverse childhood experiences can exert a negative impact on their clinical course (Gu et al. 2022; Herzog and Schmahl 2018). Negative childhood experiences can result in structural and functional changes of the brain, such as in the hippocampus and amygdala, that are associated with the development of bipolar and depressive illnesses (Cassiers et al. 2018). Somatic effects of childhood trauma can include disturbances of the stress axis and immune-inflammatory mechanisms as well as metabolic dysregulation (Jaworska-Andryszewska and Rybakowski 2019).

Mind-Body Connectedness Theories

Various nursing theories help illustrate the importance of mind-body connectedness and can inform choices for care. We summarize three of these in Table 5.1: the Adaptation Model by Roy, the Theory of Unpleasant Symptoms by Lens & Pugh, and the Theory of Symptom Management by Humphries and colleagues (see Table 5.1).

Table 5.1 Physical trauma and mental health outcomes: examples of nursing theories to inform nursing process

Theory	Theorist(s)	Central concepts/components	Nursing process steps	Considerations for application
Adaptation model	Roy	Person, health, environment, nursing	Assessment of behaviour, assessment of stimuli, diagnosis, goal-setting, goal-focused intervention, evaluation of goal attainment	A person is in constant interaction with a changing environment; this interaction requires positive adaptation to promote health; throughout the nursing process, nurses adapt the plan of care based on the patient's health progress (Roy and Andrews 1999)
Theory of Unpleasant Symptoms (TOUS)	Lens and Pugh	Symptoms (patient-perceived changes in normal functioning)	Importance of assessing multiple symptoms occurring simultaneously	Focuses on managing multiple symptoms that may occur at the same time; is inclusive of physical, psychological, situational and environmental factors' influence and interplay on symptoms (Mary Jane Smith and Liehr 2018)—Chap. 8
Theory of Symptom Management (SMT)	Humphries et al.	Symptom experience, symptom management strategies, symptom status outcomes	Assess symptoms, develop and implement effective management strategies, evaluate outcomes	Symptom experience varies by person, environment, and health/illness; individuals' symptom perception is affected by awareness of symptoms, initiation of management strategies, and assessment of symptom outcomes (Mary Jane Smith and Liehr 2018)—Chap. 7

Possible Sources of Trauma and Response

SAMHSA has proposed a "3 E" model (Fig. 5.4) that can be used to categorize traumatic encounters into factors related to the Event, the Experience of the event, or the predicted severity of the Effects (Lathan et al. 2021; SAMHSA 2014).

Fig. 5.4 SAMHSA "3 E" model

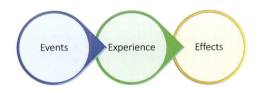

Event

The consequences of interpersonal trauma, from one person to another (e.g. physical abuse, sexual assault, intimate partner violence), may be interpreted or internalized differently than those of non-interpersonal trauma (natural weather events; vehicular accidents) (Kessler et al. 2017). Interpersonal trauma often interrupts an individual's foundational beliefs and can contribute towards more complex outcomes. The number of different traumas experienced has been found to be predictive of symptom complexity compared to a single traumatic event (Kessler et al. 2017).

Experience

How the individual appraises their experience of trauma can directly influence their process of recovery. A sense of betrayal and violation often contributes to significant physical, psychological, and relational distress.

Effect

There are multiple clinical diagnoses related to trauma experiences, as described within the Diagnostic and Statistical Manual of Mental Disorders (DSM-5 TR) (APA 2022), which relate to context, time, and age of the individuals who have experienced trauma (see Table 5.2).

Trauma-and stressor-related disorders encompass a range of conditions that develop in response to exposure to significant stress or trauma. These disorders vary in presentation but commonly involve disturbances in emotional regulation, attachment, mood, and behaviour. Table 5.3 outlines key trauma-related disorders, summarizing their core symptoms and potential outcomes. Understanding these conditions is essential for accurate diagnosis and effective intervention, ensuring appropriate support and treatment for individuals affected by traumatic experiences.

Holistic nursing interventions play a critical role in addressing the physical, emotional, and psychological needs of patients and their families following physical trauma. As shown in Fig. 5.5, these interventions prioritize physical and emotional safety, include family members and friends in the care process as appropriate, and consider legal and cultural factors to ensure comprehensive, culturally sensitive care.

5 Traumatic Physical Injuries and Mental Health Outcomes

Table 5.2 Possible physical reactions to trauma

Immediate (minutes to <1 month post-incident)	Delayed (≥1 month to years post-incident)
Nausea and/or gastrointestinal distress Sweating or shivering Faintness Muscle tremors or uncontrollable shaking Elevated heartbeat, respiration, and blood pressure Extreme fatigue or exhaustion Greater startle responses Depersonalization	Sleep disturbances, nightmares Somatization (e.g. increased focus on and worry about body aches and pains) Appetite and digestive changes Lowered resistance to colds and infection Persistent fatigue Elevated cortisol levels Hyperarousal Long-term health effects including heart, liver, autoimmune, and chronic obstructive pulmonary disease

Symptoms present and may be categorized as acute or posttraumatic depending on the time when the trauma was experienced (APA 2022)

Table 5.3 Trauma and stressor-related disorders

Disorder	Summary of symptoms	Potential outcomes
Reactive attachment disorder	The child rarely or minimally seeks or responds to comfort when distressed The child has experienced a pattern of extremes of insufficient care The child has experienced a pattern of extremes of insufficient care	Pattern of disturbed or developmentally inappropriate attachment behaviours
Disinhibited social engagement disorder	Actively approaching and interacting with unfamiliar adults with—verbal or physical behaviour, socially disinhibited behaviour, and lack of age-appropriate social boundaries	A pattern of behaviour in which a child is involved in culturally inappropriate, overly familiar, interactions with unfamiliar adults
Posttraumatic stress disorder	Behavioural symptom clusters described as re-experiencing, avoidance, negative cognitions and mood, and arousal	Development of symptoms following exposure to one or more traumatic events
Acute stress disorder	Behavioural symptoms clusters described as intrusion, negative mood, dissociation, avoidance, and arousal	Symptoms following exposure to one or more traumatic events that last 3 days up to a month post-exposure
Adjustment disorder	Distress out of proportion to the severity and intensity of the stressor Significant social or occupational or functional impairment	Emotional or behavioural symptoms in response to an identifiable stressor that lasts 3 months or more after exposure (grief is excluded)

Other specified trauma- and stressor-related disorder; unspecified trauma-and stressor-related disorder

Adapted from DSM-5-TR APA (2022)

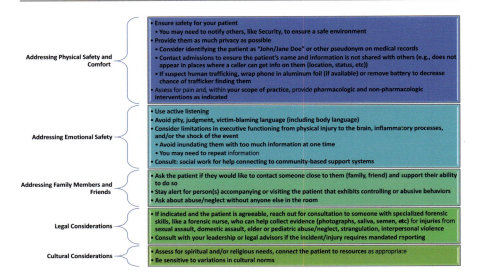

Fig. 5.5 Holistic nursing interventions for patients and families after physical trauma

Summary

Physical and psychological trauma result in a dynamic interplay between several body systems, which must be considered during all phases of the nursing process. Inflammatory processes can influence both acute and long-term symptoms. Whether trauma is reported immediately or is delayed can influence clinicians' assessment and treatment approaches. Other considerations of physical trauma should include but not be limited to presentations related to pain, blood loss, hypoxia/anoxia, cellular damage, disfigurement, and functional disability. Various theories from nursing and other disciplines, as well as frameworks from organizations like SAMHSA, can provide support for clinicians as they partner with their patients in navigating life after trauma. As appropriate, the clinician can offer opportunities for continued therapeutic follow-ups, as well as provide referrals for medication management, connection to community-based resources, physical and/or occupational therapy, neuropsychiatric testing, and cultural and religious support.

Case

Mark is an Army Master Sergeant about to retire after 20 years of service, including three tours of duty in active conflict zones. Mark's wife, Karla, reports a recent significant change in Mark's mood paired with difficulty sleeping, recurring nightmares, and no interest in attending his weekly basketball games with his friends from the Army. Mark has a history of mild traumatic brain injuries while in service and has been cleared as physically healthy.

Discussion Questions

- What factors might be influencing Mark's sudden change in behaviour?
- What might be the impact of multiple exposures to TBI events?
- What might the symptoms of Mark's behaviour be linked to?
- How could Karla contribute to his plan of care?
- What other questions could we ask Mark and Karla to get a comprehensive history?
- How would you prioritize care for Mark?

Concepts

Adverse childhood experiences
Cytokines
Epigenetic regulation
Functional deficits
HPA axis
Interpersonal trauma
Neuroinflammation
Non-interpersonal trauma
Physical trauma
Structural deficits
Sustained inflammation
Traumatic brain injury

References

APA (2022) DSM-5-TR(tm) classification. American Psychiatric Association Publishing

Balikji J, Hoogbergen MM, Garssen J, Verster JC (2022) Mental resilience, mood, and quality of life in young adults with self-reported impaired wound healing. Int J Environ Res Public Health 19(5). https://doi.org/10.3390/ijerph19052542

Breton CV, Landon R, Kahn LG, Enlow MB, Peterson AK, Bastain T et al (2021) Exploring the evidence for epigenetic regulation of environmental influences on child health across generations. Commun Biol 4(1):769. https://doi.org/10.1038/s42003-021-02316-6

Cassiers LLM, Sabbe BGC, Schmaal L, Veltman DJ, Penninx B, Van Den Eede F (2018) Structural and functional brain abnormalities associated with exposure to different childhood trauma subtypes: A systematic review of neuroimaging findings. Front Psych 9:329. https://doi.org/10.3389/fpsyt.2018.00329

Chrousos GP (2009) Stress and disorders of the stress system. Nat Rev Endocrinol 5(7):374–381. https://doi.org/10.1038/nrendo.2009.106

Gu W, Zhao Q, Yuan C, Yi Z, Zhao M, Wang Z (2022) Impact of adverse childhood experiences on the symptom severity of different mental disorders: a cross-diagnostic study. Gen Psychiatr 35(2):e100741. https://doi.org/10.1136/gpsych-2021-100741

Herrera-Escobar JP, Osman SY, Das S, Toppo A, Orlas CP, Castillo-Angeles M et al (2021) Long-term patient-reported outcomes and patient-reported outcome measures after injury: the

National Trauma Research Action Plan (NTRAP) scoping review. J Trauma Acute Care Surg 90(5):891–900. https://doi.org/10.1097/ta.0000000000003108

Herzog JI, Schmahl C (2018) Adverse childhood experiences and the consequences on neurobiological, psychosocial, and somatic conditions across the lifespan. Front Psych 9:420. https://doi.org/10.3389/fpsyt.2018.00420

Hori H, Kim Y (2019) Inflammation and post-traumatic stress disorder. Psychiatry Clin Neurosci 73(4):143–153. https://doi.org/10.1111/pcn.12820

Jaworska-Andryszewska P, Rybakowski JK (2019) Childhood trauma in mood disorders: neurobiological mechanisms and implications for treatment. Pharmacol Rep 71(1):112–120. https://doi.org/10.1016/j.pharep.2018.10.004

Jiang S, Postovit L, Cattaneo A, Binder EB, Aitchison KJ (2019) Epigenetic modifications in stress response genes associated with childhood trauma. Front Psych 10:808. https://doi.org/10.3389/fpsyt.2019.00808

Kessler RC, Aguilar-Gaxiola S, Alonso J, Benjet C, Bromet EJ, Cardoso G et al (2017) Trauma and PTSD in the WHO world mental health surveys. Eur J Psychotraumatol 8(sup5):1353383. https://doi.org/10.1080/20008198.2017.1353383

Krug EG, Mercy JA, Dahlberg LL, Zwi AB (2002) The world report on violence and health. Lancet 360(9339):1083–1088. https://doi.org/10.1016/s0140-6736(02)11133-0

Lathan EC, Selwyn CN, Langhinrichsen-Rohling J (2021) The "3 Es" of trauma-informed care in a federally qualified health center: traumatic event- and experience-related predictors of physical and mental health effects among female patients. J Community Psychol 49(2):703–724. https://doi.org/10.1002/jcop.22488

Quidé Y, Tozzi L, Corcoran M, Cannon DM, Dauvermann MR (2020) The impact of childhood trauma on developing bipolar disorder: current understanding and ensuring continued Progress. Neuropsychiatr Dis Treat 16:3095–3115. https://doi.org/10.2147/ndt.s285540

Robert S (2020) Traumatic brain injury and mood disorders. Ment Health Clin 10(6):335–345. https://doi.org/10.9740/mhc.2020.11.335

Rodney T, Osier N, Gill J (2018) Pro- and anti-inflammatory biomarkers and traumatic brain injury outcomes: A review. Cytokine 110:248–256. https://doi.org/10.1016/j.cyto.2018.01.012

Roy C, Andrews HA (1999) The Roy adaptation model. Prentice Hall

SAMHSA (2014) SAMHSA's concept of trauma and guidance for a trauma-informed approach. Retrieved from https://ncsacw.acf.hhs.gov/userfiles/files/SAMHSA_Trauma.pdf

Smith MJ, Liehr PR (2018) Middle range theory for nursing, 4th edn. Springer Publishing Company

Thumfart KM, Jawaid A, Bright K, Flachsmann M, Mansuy IM (2022) Epigenetics of childhood trauma: long term sequelae and potential for treatment. Neurosci Biobehav Rev 132:1049–1066. https://doi.org/10.1016/j.neubiorev.2021.10.042

Trauma Experience and the Impact on Caregivers in Formal and Family Settings: Ethical Considerations

Georgina Morley and Louise Isham

Objectives
- To describe the concepts of moral distress, compassion fatigue, and vicarious trauma
- To identify the impact of caring for patients who have experienced trauma on formal carers (healthcare workers) and family carers
- To describe the ethical considerations and differences between formal and family carers

Introduction

The principal focus of this book is the ways in which healthcare providers can identify and meet the needs of people who have experienced different forms of trauma. This chapter adopts a divergent but complementary perspective by (1) exploring the ethical obligations of nurses and (2) the ethical implications and often hidden costs to caregivers of witnessing and supporting people who are traumatized and managing personal experiences of trauma. To this end, this chapter explores a range of key concepts, such as 'vicarious trauma', 'moral distress', and 'compassion fatigue' (see Table 6.1 for details). Seeking to understand how caring in the context of trauma feels, looks, and is made sense of, the chapter considers critically how existing research and theory about how working in challenging environments may shape

---

G. Morley (✉)
Center for Bioethics & Stanley S. Zielony Institute for Nursing Excellence, Cleveland Clinic, Cleveland, OH, USA
e-mail: morleyg@ccf.org

L. Isham
Department of Social Work and Social Care, University of Birmingham, Birmingham, UK
e-mail: l.j.isham@bham.ac.uk

© The Author(s), under exclusive license to Springer Nature Switzerland AG 2025
T. Rodney (ed.), *Trauma Informed Care*,
https://doi.org/10.1007/978-3-031-87526-7_6

Table 6.1 Sub-categories of moral distress[a]

Moral distress sub-category	Description
Moral-conflict distress	The moral agent experiences psychological distress that is caused because they are engaged in conflict with another moral agent about the most ethically appropriate action
Moral-constraint distress	The moral agent experiences psychological distress that is caused because they are constrained from doing what they think or believe to be the most appropriate ethical action
Moral-tension distress	The moral agent experiences psychological distress that is caused because they feel unable to share their beliefs with others
Moral-dilemma distress	The moral agent experiences psychological distress that is caused because they are unable to choose between two or more moral requirements
Moral-uncertainty distress	The moral agent experiences psychological distress that is caused because they feel uncertain about the most ethically appropriate action

[a]Adapted from Morley et al. (2022); Morley et al. (2020b)

(and limit) the way trauma is identified and responded to in formal and family settings. Conventionally, there is a separation between formal carers, those who have a paid, professional role, such as nurses, and so-called 'informal' carers, i.e., people who care within intimate and family relationships. This chapter considers both groups and seeks to trouble the demarcation between them.

In the first part of this chapter, two different ethical theories are described: care ethics and feminist ethics. These ethical theories will be applied to nursing practice to illuminate nurses' ethical responsibilities to patients. Underpinned by feminist ethics of care, caring is conceptualized as encompassing both the actions and tasks involved in attending to another person's intimate or healthcare needs as well as recognizing care as an expression of relational and ethical responsibilities often underpinned by feelings of compassion, consideration, and responsibility (Forbat 2005; Barnes 2012). To overcome some of the noted deficiencies in care ethics, consideration of feminist bioethics will also be integrated with issues of power and justice in relation to formal and family caregiving.

Looking at the different ways that trauma is identified and responded to in formal and family care contexts helps to surface the different ways that 'types' of caregivers are imagined and prioritized, which in turn leads to differences in training, support, and social recognition. These considerations are explored by following two patients who have experienced different types of trauma, from acute hospital admission to discharge into their home setting. This will provide the settings for us to explore the impact of trauma on both formal and family caregivers.

Ethical Theories

Ethics concerns what is 'good', 'right', or 'best' and encompasses questions about how to live a good life and what we 'ought' to do (Beauchamp and Childress 2013; Johnstone 2009). Bioethics is the study of ethical, social, and legal issues that arise in biomedicine and biomedical research. Often, the terms 'ethics' and 'bioethics' are used interchangeably in the healthcare setting. There are a number of different ethical theories that provide frameworks for determining the 'right' or 'least bad' pathway. A brief overview of common ethical theories is provided in Box 6.1. Most nursing curricula will teach nurses and other healthcare students 'Principlism', which draws upon the use of ethical principles for moral decision-making. Most frequently, nurses and others are taught the four principles of biomedical ethics (see Box 6.1). However, these principles can come into conflict, and we need to draw upon the particulars of the situation to identify the ethically acceptable pathways forward. Furthermore, the four principles do not nurture consideration of the relational aspects of care that are so important to nursing and which will be central to this chapter.

Care Ethics

Care ethics developed from the work of Gilligan (1982) and Noddings (1984) in response to the work of Kohlberg (1981). Kohlberg (1981), a moral psychologist, conducted research with boys aged 10–16 to gain an understanding of moral development. Kohlberg developed a series of moral dilemmas that were presented to male adolescent research participants who were asked in an interview to explain their thinking when resolving a moral dilemma. From these findings, Kohlberg (1981) argued that there are three stages of moral development, each with two sub-stages: pre-conventional (pre-moral), conventional and post-conventional (principled morality). At each of these levels, Kohlberg suggests that the individual is exhibiting moral reasoning, which culminates in the final stage, which is the ability to utilize abstract moral principles within one's reasoning. In the sixth stage, the individual is able to use a 'deontological' approach to ethics in which moral requirements and moral prohibitions are justified based upon the value of the action in itself, rather than the consequences of those actions (see Box 6.1 for a description of deontology). Kohlberg grounded this sixth stage in a Kantian approach to morality in which universal 'maxims' or moral rules guide action. Kohlberg suggested that while men were concerned with striving for justice and autonomy for individuals within society, women would not reach this sixth stage of moral development.

Gilligan (1982) rejected Kohlberg's theory and conclusions and conducted her own empirical work with women. Gilligan (1982) argued that women and men resolve moral problems differently, suggesting that women are more concerned with honouring relationships than fulfilling ethical principles and rules. As Kohlen (2020) describes,

> Their [Gilligan's] moral reflections revealed the relevance of a contextual understanding… She concluded that human beings live their life in a network of dependence and contrasted the voice of care with the voice of justice. The voice of care is seen as a moral orientation that pays attention to the particularities of individual situations and the meaning of relationships as an integral part of moral judgement. (p. 122)

Gilligan identified that caring was central to the way in which women approached moral thinking and structured a theory of caring as parallel to Kohlberg's three stages: pre-caring, transcaring (which is bound by roles and rules), and person-centred caring (McLeod-Sordjan 2014).

Noddings (1984) was also highly influential in the development of an ethics of care, but in contrast to Gilligan, Noddings focused on caring as a practical activity. Noddings (2002) highlights how individuals are not born as rational, isolated decision-makers but instead are born as vulnerable beings in need of caring by others. Noddings (1984) distinguished between the caregiver and care-receiver and stressed that this is not a paternal relationship in which the caregiver subordinates the care-receiver's needs but a reciprocal relationship. The caregiver identifies and attends to the needs of the care-receiver, responding to them as best they are able given the resources and conditions (Noddings 2002). In return, the care-receiver recognizes the efforts of the caregiver, and if this is not forthcoming, then according to Noddings (2002), it is not truly a 'caring' relationship. Recognition need not be through gratitude but simply acknowledging that care has been received.

Noddings (2015) suggests that caring is 'needs' based and contrasts this to justice, that is 'rights' based, anchored in individual rights and duties. Noddings (2015) argues that needs (or wants) are more basic than rights and that needs become rights once individuals can exercise power to satisfy their needs. It seems that for this reason, Noddings (2015) argues that care ethics is both 'broader' and 'deeper' than feminist ethics (p. 73). Noddings (2015) quotes Virginia Held:

> Care is probably the most deeply fundamental value. There can be care without justice: There has historically been little justice in the family, but care and life have gone on without it. There can be no justice without care, however, for without care no child would survive and there would be no persons to respect. (2005, 17)

Feminist ethicists have however critiqued care ethics and the work of Noddings and Gilligan. Bringing Noddings care ethics into the clinical realm, Kuhse (1997) critiques Nodding's notion of caring as 'engrossment'. Kuhse (1997) argues that there is 'a great danger in requiring that every nurse–patient encounter be a "total encounter" and in thus setting the ideal of caring in nursing too high' (p. 149). She questions whether this is even something that all patients would want: 'It seems highly unlikely that every patient who enters hospital with a particular medical problem—say, to have her appendix or her varicose veins removed—would *want* the many different nurses who look after her during her hospitalisation to make serious efforts to "enter her life space"' (p. 149). Indeed, the expectation of nurses to form an intimate connection with all their patients in such a way seems to ask too much of both the nurse and the patient. If we consider this within the context of trauma, in which a patient might be dealing with a life-altering illness or injury, then we might question the utility of this form of caring and whether it might be determined to be too intimate or intense. The formation of boundaries for both the caregiver and receiver may be required and indeed healthy in many circumstances. It is also not entirely clear how a relationship of 'engrossment' would necessarily ensure ethical care.

Scholars have also argued that Gilligan's dichotomy between the way in which men and women approach moral thinking exacerbates gender divides and the gender binary. From an intersectional perspective, Gilligan failed to recruit participants from different racial and socioeconomic backgrounds and interviewed only white, middle-upper-class women. Recruitment of diverse participants within research continues to be a problem and perpetuates the development of theories that fail to incorporate the experiences and considerations of underrepresented and minoritized individuals, thereby preventing whole populations from experiencing the benefits of research. From a feminist ethics perspective, Noddings and care ethics have generally been criticized for failing to account for the issue of justice and power. Women continue to make up the largest proportion of nurses and care workers and are frequently inadequately remunerated or recognized within these professions. Women are also more likely to take on unpaid caring roles in family care settings, taking on care of children, elder care, and loved ones experiencing illness. This work is frequently hidden and unrecognized within society. Unlike feminist ethics, it is less clear how care ethics provides a position from which these social and political issues can be critiqued and called to attention. Jaggar (2001) famously stated that 'femin*ine* is not necessarily femin*ist*' (p. 532) because more is required from a feminist response than simply drawing divides between genders.

Feminist Ethics

Care ethics and feminist ethics both stand in stark contrast to 'traditional' moral philosophy and the ethical theories therein (see Box 6.1 for a brief description of some common ethical theories).

As described by Gotlib (2022),

> feminist ethical theory can be understood as both a response to, and a movement against, a historical tradition of more abstract, universalist, ethical theories such as utilitarianism, deontology, and in certain respects, contractarianism and virtue theory, which tend to view the moral agent either as an autonomous, rational actor, deliberating out of a calculus of utility or duty, or else as an often disembodied and decontextualized ideal decision-maker, unburdened by the non-ideal constraints of luck (moral and otherwise), circumstance, or capability.

Both care ethics and feminist ethics stipulate that our relationships, responsibilities, and social and political positions ('positionality') in the world are of central importance. Though arguably, as touched upon in the previous section, critics of care ethics would argue that care ethics fails to sufficiently account for women's social and political positions, arguing 'caring' is not enough, that we need to be able to uphold standards of justice (Card 1990; Nelson 1992). We explore some of the deficits of care ethics in contrast to feminist ethics later in this chapter when we discuss the impact of caring on family caregivers. In this section, we provide a high-level overview of feminist ethics.

Feminist ethicists and philosophers have sought to highlight the ways in which traditional moral philosophy has devalued women and marginalized individuals' experiences, idealizing notions of universality and rationality in moral decision-making and minimizing the role of emotion and responsibility. This does not require that feminist ethicists reject all previous ethical theories but rather that they seek to expand the scope and nature of ethical inquiry, drawing attention to those who are marginalized within society, such as women, Black, Indigenous and People of Colour, and LGBTQIA+ individuals. As Jaggar (1991) argues, moral principles (such as those found in Principlism—see Box 6.1) are interpreted differently in various contexts and societies and, therefore, generate different conclusions about right and wrong. Consider, for example, that individuals in some contexts articulate the belief that there is value in experiencing some level of pain at the end of life. This directly conflicts with Western norms of relieving pain and suffering at death, which uphold ethical principles of beneficence and non-maleficence. Jaggar (1991) states that 'it is increasingly accepted that reason is culturally constituted, consisting primarily of sets of traditional practices that take various forms' (p. 93). This grounds moral knowing in moral experience that is 'plural and local rather than singular and universal, grounded not in transcendent reason' (p. 93). Jaggar (1991) argues that this perspective does not commit feminists to moral relativism, which is the view that moral judgements are true or false relative only to a particular standpoint (Westacott 2022). All intersectional feminist ethicists will always object to the subordination of women and marginalized individuals in any setting, context, or culture.

This may beg the question then, how do feminist ethicists make moral determinations or make moral decisions? As Jaggar (1991) suggests, feminist ethicists do not need to be committed to one particular ethical theory and may build upon a number of various approaches, principles, or norms to reach decisions. However, feminists are committed to valuing women's and minoritized individuals experiences, seeking to overcome power imbalances, and striving for equality and justice. Walker (2007) coins her approach to morality an 'expressive-collaborative model' which she positions in contrast to the 'theoretical-judicial model' of traditional moral philosophy (as can be found in deontological approaches—see Box 6.1) which presents 'morality as a compact, propositionally codifiable, impersonally action-guiding code' employed by a rational 'well-formed moral agent' (p. 8). Walker's (2007) expressive-collaborative model instead positions ethics as socially, historically, and politically constructed. It requires continuous negotiation between individuals living in a community:

> The theoretical-judicial model pictured morality as an individual action-guiding system within or for a person. The expressive-collaborative conception pictures morality as a socially embodied medium of understanding and adjustment in which people account to each other for identities, relationships, and values that define their responsibilities. (pp. 67–68)

This requires understanding the narrative and context of people's lives, the relationships that are most important to them, and the responsibilities that they feel compelled to uphold and maintain. To reach a moral decision or understanding, this narrative will also include shared norms, maxims, principles, and guidelines. Significantly for this chapter, this will look different in the professional setting of caregiving and the family setting.

Box 6.1: Ethical Theories

Deontological Ethics: Deontological theories hold that some moral choices are morally forbidden and cannot be determined to be right or wrong based upon their consequences. Kant (1724–1804) is one of the most known deontologists, recognized for developing the 'categorical imperative' which stipulates that one should only carry out an action if that action should be universalized, meaning everyone could 'will' it to be a 'universal law'. The categorical imperative states, 'act only in accordance with that maxim through which you can at the same time will that it become a universal law' (Korsgaard 1997).

Principlism: Principlism is a deontological approach to moral decision-making that draws upon *prima facie* (meaning 'on the face of it' or true unless proven otherwise) ethical principles to guide ethical analysis and to provide justification for normative recommendations. The 'Principles of Biomedical Ethics' by Beauchamp and Childress (2015) is a seminal and influential text in which they describe in depth the following four principles: respect for autonomy, beneficence, non-maleficence, and justice.

Consequentialism: Consequentialist ethical theories are often referred to as 'teleological', derived from the Greek teleos, meaning 'end' and are often contrasted with deontological theories. This approach to ethical analysis is concerned with the consequences of actions rather than the value of the action itself. For example, stealing food in order to feed a starving child could be justified based upon the good consequences of the bad action.

Utilitarianism: Utilitarianism is a consequentialist ethical theory because the justification of the action is based upon the consequences. However, in utilitarianism, the individual should identify morally preferable actions by considering which action maximizes utility or happiness for the greatest number. Utilitarianism can be divided into two different types: act and rule. Act Utilitarians stipulate that in order to judge whether an action should be carried out, it should be judged based upon whether it will provide the greatest net benefit. Whereas Rule Utilitarians consider whether an action conforms to a justified moral rule, and a moral rule is only justified if it creates more utility than other rules.

Virtue Ethics: Virtue ethics holds that virtue and character are central to ethical behaviour. Originally developed by Aristotle (384–322 B.C.), a Greek philosopher, and later revived by Anscombe (1958) and MacIntyre (1981). There are a number of virtue-based approaches to ethics in which it is argued that morality should move away from a legalistic, principles-based theory to valuing the development of good moral character.

Ethical Responsibilities in the Formal and Family Care Settings

The responsibilities that nurses and other healthcare professionals uphold are governed by professional standards such as providing care that is evidence-based and are bound by their professional code of ethics. Whereas, a partner caring for their loved one in the home is not held to the same kinds of professional standards, though continue to be governed by societal and ethical norms.

The content of nurses' professional code of ethics varies between countries. There is, however, also an international code of ethics produced by the International Council of Nurses (ICN 2021), which was recently revised in 2021. The ICN states that this is not supposed to be a 'code of conduct' but rather a framework to guide ethical nursing practice and decision-making that meets professional standards set forth by regulators. The ICN Code of Ethics consists of four elements (see Box 6.2), and in each element, there are a set of statements such as 'Nurses advocate for equity and social justice in resource allocation, access to health care and other social and economic services' (p. 7). At the end of each section, the ICN provides a brief example of how nurses, nurse leaders, educators, researchers, and national nursing associations might uphold each element.

By contrast, the American Nurses Association Code of Ethics for Nurses (2025) consists of ten provisions, each of which contains specific statements that elucidate the way in which these provisions can be applied. Fowler (2016) argues that the ANA Code of Ethics for Nurses demonstrates nursing's long commitment to a social ethics that aims to address the social determinants of health and unjust social structures, thus echoing some of the concerns of feminist ethics described in the previous section (see Box 6.2).

Box 6.2: Core Commitments in the ICN and ANA Code of Ethics and the NMC Code of Conduct

Four elements in the International Council of Nurses Code of Ethics (2021)	Ten provisions in the American Nurses Association Code of Ethics for Nurses (2025)	Four standards of conduct or behaviour in the Nursing and Midwifery Council Code of Conduct (2015)
1. Nurses and patients or other people requiring care or services. 2. Nurses and practice. 3. Nurses and the profession. 4. Nurses and global health.	1. The nurse practices with compassion and respect for the inherent dignity, worth, and unique attributes of every person. 2. A nurse's primary commitment is to the recipient(s) of nursing care, whether an individual, family, group, community, or population. 3. The nurse establishes a trusting relationship and advocates for the rights, health, and safety of recipient(s) of nursing care. 4. Nurses have authority over nursing practice and are responsible and accountable for their practice consistent with their obligations to promote health, prevent illness, and provide optimal care. 5. The nurse has moral duties to self as a person of inherent dignity and worth, including an expectation of a safe place to work that fosters flourishing, authenticity of self at work, and self-respect through integrity and professional competence. 6. Nurses, through individual and collective effort, establish, maintain, and improve the ethical environment of the work setting that affects nursing care and the well-being of nurses. 7. Nurses advance the profession through multiple approaches to knowledge development, professional standards, and the generation of policies for nursing, health, and social concerns. 8. Nurses build collaborative relationships and networks with nurses, other healthcare and nonhealthcare disciplines, and the public to achieve greater ends. 9. Nurses and their professional organizations work to enact and resource practices, policies, and legislation to promote social justice, eliminate health inequities, and facilitate human flourishing. 10. Nursing, through organizations and associations, participates in the global nursing and health community to promote human and environmental health, well-being, and flourishing.	1. Prioritize people. 2. Practice effectively. 3. Preserve safety. 4. Promote professionalism and trust.

The ANA Code of Ethics for Nurses (2025) reflects a more detailed guidance when compared to the ICN Code of Ethics (2021), and the United Kingdom's Nursing and Midwifery Council (NMC 2015) Code of Conduct in providing ethical guidance to nurses. The strength of the ANA Code of Ethics for Nurses is in the interpretive statements that elucidate each statement. However, as Snelling (2016) highlights, a code of ethics by no means exhaustively captures all of a nurse's professional responsibilities. Rather, they summarize core standards that nurses ought to uphold to the extent possible in complex circumstances and provide insight for the public regarding what they should expect of nurses. As Snelling (2016) states, there are distinct differences between codes of conduct (e.g. the NMC Code) and ethical theories and principles (e.g. virtue ethics). They are intertwined in important ways since codes of conduct draw upon ethical ideals, but it is also important to recognize that Codes are regulatory requirements, which suggests that each statement can and should be fulfilled. Whereas within ethics, it is well recognized that ethical principles and commitments often come into conflict. As Snelling (2016) states,

> Like the law, conduct-rules tell us what we must do and what we must not do, and while it is also the case that ethical-rules also set out the obligatory and the forbidden, they are additionally concerned with what is permissible or justified or aspired to. Both sets of rules have a role in education and regulation, but clarity is required so that they can be distinguished. This necessarily requires precision with language, and regulators do not always provide it. (p. 239)

The ANA Code of Ethics for Nurses provides a code that is not only deontological in terms of providing rule-like statements, such as the nurse *must* be knowledgeable about advanced directive documents, but also provides descriptive, normative statements such as nurses *should* provide care that is sensitive to diverse cultural values.

Reflection Point
- After reviewing Box 6.2, what do you think are the common and shared elements between each of the codes of ethics/codes of conduct?
- Review the code of ethics or code of conduct that applies to you and think about how it guides your behaviour as a professional nurse. Do you think that codes of ethics are sufficient for providing ethical guidance? Do you think there needs to be additional ethics support for nurses?

Application of Care Ethics and Feminist Ethics to Nursing Practice

Both care ethics and feminist ethics have great applicability to nursing practice, and many nursing ethics scholars have utilized care ethics and feminist ethics to inform their conceptual and empirical work. Fry (1989) argues that traditional 'masculine' approaches to medical ethics do not provide an appropriate model for nursing ethics because it relies upon the four principles (Principlism) and the context for justification, rather than the context within which decisions are taking place. Drawing on care ethics, Fry (1989) argues that caring ought to be a foundational value for nursing ethics. Fry (1989) highlights a number of different scholars' proposals for the way in which caring might provide a moral foundation for nursing ethics:

- Gadow (1985) suggests that truth-telling and touch might form the basis of ethical nursing actions. Truth-telling provides the basis of decision-making with the nurse assisting to contextualize decisions in terms of patients lived experiences of their illness. The role of touch enables the nurse to help the patient to feel valued.
- Watson (1985) suggests that the preservation of humanity and the promotion of dignity might form the foundations of a caring ideal foundational to nursing practice.
- Frankena (1983) suggests a moral point-of-view approach that requires adopting a particular moral value or principle (such as caring) and then taking a general stance from which to begin normative theorizing.

Fry (1989) suggests that these approaches may contribute to robust nursing ethics but does not elucidate on exactly what a nursing ethics framework might be. Fry and Johnstone (2002) later suggest that a theory of nursing ethics would intertwine virtue ethics, nursing heritage, and nursing codes of ethics. Fry states:

> The 'good' nurse of the 21st century will be a composite ideal shaped by empirical evidence about the ethical reality of nurses' practices and by the ethical standards for nursing practice set forth by organizations such as ICN [International Council of Nurses]. (Fry and Johnstone 2002, p. 2)

McCarthy (2006) critiques the notion that there ought to be a separate and distinct theory of nursing ethics. McCarthy's (2006) key objections are that a separate and distinct theory would fail to capture the diverse nature of nursing practice, the differences and similarities between nurses and their ethical obligations to patients and families, and would require that one singular ethical framework have applicability between different ethical questions and contexts. McCarthy (2006) instead suggests that nursing ethics should take a pluralist (the position that many ethical theories have value and truth) and a critical stance towards existing ethical frameworks. This approach to nursing ethics could draw upon any one of the ethical theories that have been mentioned so far in this chapter to provide justification for action.

On this approach, a nurse identifying the ethically supportable pathways might draw upon the principle of beneficence to identify how they might act to promote the patient's conception of a good outcome, while also considering the most important relationships within that patients' life, working to involve those loved ones in the decision-making or caregiving process, and mitigating to the extent able any power wielded over the patient in the decision-making process. As McCarthy (2006) highlights, the quality of decision-making depends a lot on both moral reasoning skills and a fair and just process:

> The features of good decision-making include: awareness of the socio-political context, sensitivity to the moral dimensions of the situation, conceptual clarity, imaginative and rigorous argumentation, critical evaluation of theoretical presuppositions… the Pluralist View acknowledges that making ethical decisions is often messy and heart wrenching business and that our finest ethical decisions are not those about which we are certain; they are those with which we can live and which prompt us to do better next time. (p. 163)

In the rest of this chapter, two case studies are explored through the lens of care ethics and feminist ethics, recognizing that caring for others is a central activity of human flourishing while also calling to attention considerations of power and marginalization in these caring relationships.

Working in the Context of Trauma: Exploring the Impact on Professional Caregivers

Over the past three decades, recognizing the physical, emotional, and psychological impact on caregivers of working in intimate, challenging, and often unpredictable situations has grown. Grounded in the experiences of nurses and nursing organizations, some of the insights generated from research and theory can help us to understand the benefits and costs of caring in a trauma-informed way (Isobel and Thomas 2022). To understand the impact of nursing in contexts of trauma, it is first important to outline what caregiving can 'look' and 'feel' like. That is, to understand the environments and spaces in which nursing care can take place, as well as the ethical and emotional standards expected of nurses, as set by their professional bodies, employing organizations, and wider social factors. The case studies of Jerome and Frances provide context to the concepts described in this chapter.

In the following section, three ways of understanding and explaining the impact on nurses of working in emotionally intense and potentially traumatic environments are explored: moral distress, compassion fatigue, and vicarious trauma.

Moral Distress

Moral distress was first described by Jameton (1984) as arising 'when one knows the right thing to do, but institutional constraints make it nearly impossible to pursue the right course of action' (p. 6). Jameton (1984), an American philosopher, had spoken with nurses and was struck by the distress they described because of the bureaucratic hospital systems they were required to navigate through the course of their work. Jameton (1984) claimed that nurses most frequently encountered three different ethical challenges: moral distress, moral uncertainty, and moral dilemmas. Moral dilemmas arise when there are two or more morally supportable pathways, but all involve a moral loss (Gowans 1987). For example, nurse A might feel guilt and regret because they feel obligated to prevent harm to a patient, and yet they are obligated to suction their tracheal tube and obtain daily blood samples. The nurse recognizes that the patient stated the wish to continue life-sustaining treatments unless they are regarded to be in a terminal condition. By following the patient's wishes to continue life-sustaining treatments, the nurse is arguably doing the right thing, however this does not cancel out the nurse's obligation to prevent harm and suffering, resulting in nurse A experiencing this as a moral dilemma (Tessman 2015). Moral uncertainty occurs when one is uncertain or unable to decide which value to prioritize. For example, if nurse A did not know that the patient had stated their wish to continue life-sustaining treatments, then they might be uncertain about whether to prioritize life extension or the prevention of further harm.

Jameton (1984) seemed to suggest that moral distress cannot occur when an individual is faced with a moral dilemma or experiencing moral uncertainty, and so Jameton's original definition of moral distress has been critiqued as too narrow (Campbell et al. 2016; Fourie 2015). Broadly speaking, there are now two groups of scholars: those who argue for a broader understanding of moral distress (Morley et al. 2020a, 2021b), and those who argue that moral distress is a 'term of art' and Jameton's original conceptualization should be preserved (Epstein et al. 2016).

Morley et al. (2020a, b) argue that moral distress should be understood more broadly as the psychological distress that is causally related to a moral event and then sub-categorized into five types of moral distress (see Table 6.1). Morley et al. (2020a, b) argue that a broader definition of moral distress should be adopted for the following reasons:

- 'Terms of art' should be refined when there is sufficient evidence to do so.
- Suggesting that moral distress only occurs when an individual 'knows' the right thing to do risks shutting down moral discussion and deliberation.
- Suggesting that moral distress only occurs when an individual 'knows' the right thing to do risks exacerbating feelings of anger and frustration.
- There are other moral causes of distress.
- Emphasizing the distress that arises when individuals are morally uncertain promotes moral dialogue and an understanding of different moral perspectives.
- By sub-categorizing moral distress into different types, there is the potential to be more precise about the cause of distress.

There is limited empirical literature that describes to what extent the causes of moral distress might be regarded as different or distinct in emergency or trauma settings. Wolf et al. (2016a) conducted focus groups with 17 emergency nurses to explore the nature of moral distress. They found that nurses described the challenges that occurred due to the nature of their practice environment, describing it as a 'dysfunctional practice arena' (p. 40). They described challenges related to short staffing, patient volume, and risks to the quality of care. All of these causes have been described in other practice areas as causes of moral distress. We suggest that the heightened uncertainty about diagnosis and prognosis could create greater moral uncertainty, and exposure to risk without proper safety mechanisms could create additional constraints. As Wolf et al. (2016b) discuss, nurses must balance the duty to treat with the duty to self. Also, in emergency settings, decisions about which obligation to prioritize must be made rapidly and may exacerbate moral distress.

Moral distress is a complex concept, and in recent years, there has been an increasing focus on identifying interventions or support services that can mitigate the negative effects of moral distress. It is important to note that the goal is not to eradicate moral distress entirely since it is now more widely accepted as a natural response to situations in which there are values at stake (Tigard 2018). Rather, the aim is to mitigate the negative effects such as burnout, persistent negative emotional states, and intention to leave areas of nursing that are particularly stressful and, in some cases, to leave the profession entirely.

Burnout is a concept that is interrelated with moral distress. While some researchers have suggested that moral distress is a root cause of moral distress, Kok et al. (2021) recently concluded that one's work and home stressors may also contribute. Burnout is an intense form of occupational stress that may result in somebody being emotionally or physically unable to perform some or all aspects of their role and is characterized by emotional exhaustion, depersonalization, and feeling a lack of accomplishment (Maslach et al. 1997). Any worker is at risk of burnout, though it has been well-documented in healthcare. In nursing, high workload, low staffing levels, long shifts, and a low sense of control are associated with burnout, but Dall'Ora et al. (2020) argue that more research needs to be conducted to evidence the association between burnout and nurse turnover.

Turning back to moral distress, recent literature reviews have identified a range of approaches to tackling moral distress: mindfulness, yoga, debriefing, self-reflection, narrative writing, multidisciplinary meetings, empowerment programmes, and ethics education (Imbulana et al. 2021; Morley et al. 2021a). In two reviews, authors highlighted concerns regarding methodological quality and high risk of bias, which resulted in challenges determining an effective intervention (Imbulana et al. 2021; Morley et al. 2021a), but Morley et al. (2021a) and Amos and Epstein (2022) both suggested that ethics education appeared to be a promising approach.

One way to approach moral distress might be to consider interventions and support services that are tailored to address the moral event causing the distress, as well as those designed to support the psychological distress. Morley et al. (2021c) provide a moral distress model that they suggest can be used to inform strategies and interventions, and they provide a number of recommendations to address moral distress based upon the moral distress model (Fig. 6.1). The recommendations range from establishing clinical ethics support services, establishing unit cultures that are open to nurses' perspectives, to ensuring that nurses who are in side rooms with patients who provoke feelings of moral distress are given adequate breaks and support.

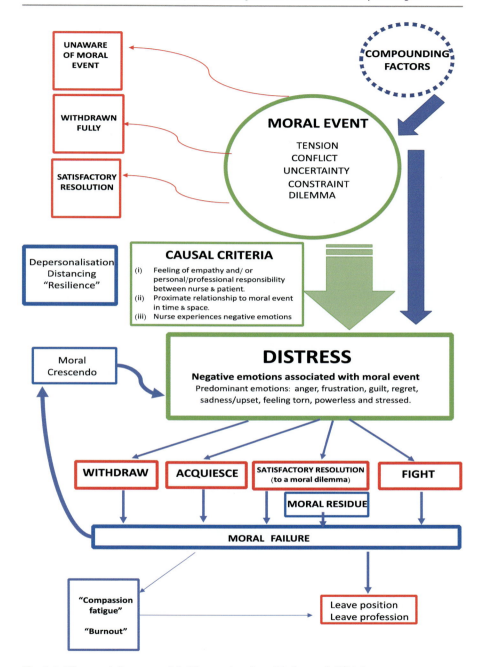

Fig. 6.1 The moral distress model. (Figure taken from Morley et al. 2021a)

In case study one, we describe three different sub-types of moral distress (moral-constraint distress, moral-uncertainty distress, and moral-tension distress) that arise for formal caregivers when they care for Jerome.

> **Case Study One: Jerome**
>
> Jerome is in his late 30s and has been hospitalized a number of times because of ingesting a foreign object; most frequently, he ingests pencils and razors. Jerome has described to his healthcare team that when he swallows an object, he is overcome with an urge or impulse and is not able to stop himself. Jerome tells his doctors that he is not trying to end his life. Jerome's healthcare team thinks that the impulse disorder is a result of his childhood trauma. Jerome is back in the critical care unit, where he has been admitted three times this month for ingestion. Jerome has to be admitted to the critical care area because the other units do not have sufficient staffing to continuously monitor him for signs of bleeding and to prevent him from swallowing another object while hospitalized.
>
> Members of the nursing team experience a range of emotions when caring for Jerome. Some of the nurses question whether the resources that are being utilized for Jerome are justified. They express anger and frustration associated with moral-constraint distress due to the lack of community and mental health resources available for Jerome. They express the feeling that it is unjust that they are using acute care resources for Jerome when his mental health disorder would be much better managed as an outpatient. Other clinicians express feeling torn, exhibiting signs of moral-uncertainty distress because they question whether they are continuing to do the right thing for Jerome. In particular, they question whether they are really making his life better by continuing to retrieve the objects he has swallowed because the lack of outpatient therapies means that when Jerome leaves the hospital, the psychological distress that he experiences is not being addressed. The clinicians also question whether they should continue endoscopic retrieval because they are concerned that his quality of life is so poor.
>
> Because of Jerome's impulse disorder, he has a healthcare assistant assigned to sit with him each day. Mary has been a healthcare assistant for ten years, and although she enjoys her job, she dislikes sitting with Jerome. When she is responsible for sitting with Jerome, she feels scared throughout her entire shift. Jerome is known to become violent within a few minutes, and it is very difficult to de-escalate him. Mary does not blame Jerome for his violent outbursts, but she does not feel that she has sufficient training and education to really manage Jerome's behaviour when he becomes agitated. Like many of the other clinicians, Mary feels unsure about whether they are really doing the right thing for Jerome, but she feels unable to share her beliefs with her colleagues, suggesting she is experiencing moral-tension distress.

More research is needed to understand the types of interventions that are most effective to mitigate the negative effects of moral distress, but it is likely that multimodal, complex interventions—and greater sociological understanding—are required to address this subjective phenomenon. In addition, there needs to be continued conceptual clarity in clinical practice and research regarding the terms and concepts we use. Conceptual clarity can help individuals to better understand causes of distress and guide the implementation of changes or interventions to address psychological distress. In the next section, the causes and consequences of trauma will be further explored through the concepts of compassion fatigue and vicarious trauma.

Compassion Fatigue

Over the past three decades, compassion fatigue has become a well-established concept among 'helping' professions such as therapists, social workers, and nurses. Compassion fatigue is predicated on people being required to behave compassionately, i.e., to be sensitive to the feelings of others and to work towards relieving their suffering. In this way, compassion fatigue differs from vicarious trauma because, regarding the latter, there is no professional (or implicit) expectation for the affected person to be engaged in some form of emotional work. However, compassion fatigue also tends to be associated with compassionate practices that take place in a professional context. As a result, the concept is rarely used to understand the experiences of family caregivers (Lynch and Lobo 2012). Compassion fatigue is broadly defined as a combination of physical and emotional exhaustion experienced by people who are expected to act in a compassionate way towards others, often in the context of caring for, or supporting people who are ill or traumatized (Peters 2018). Compassion fatigue tends to be seen as the result of behaving compassionately for a sustained period of time, or in emotionally intensive or demanding circumstances, rather than the result of 'one off' exposure to a traumatic event or situation (Lynch and Lobo 2012). Figley (2013) suggests that the concept is more agreeable to nurses than the terms 'burnout' or 'vicarious trauma' because compassion is seen as a cornerstone of nursing practice. Ledoux (2015) and Sinclair et al. (2017) also attribute the 'iconic' status of compassion as being a major driver for the interest in compassion fatigue. Most nurses understand compassion to be both an ethical value and a personal resource as well as something that can be constrained and depleted, thus developing an intuitive sense of what it means to feel 'fatigued'.

Initial manifestations of compassion fatigue include a sense of disconnectedness or withdrawal, particularly from the emotional intimacies of caring or compassionate-intensive work; over time, this can result in a more profound sense of disassociation as well as physical symptoms, such as insomnia, headaches, and conditions related to a compromised immune system (Peters 2018). If a person experiences long-term compassion fatigue, they may find it hard to sustain their caring role, with associated feelings of guilt, anxiety, and stress, and this may result in them choosing to leave their job (and in some cases, their profession) (Kelly et al. 2015). However, somebody with compassion fatigue may also find it difficult to initially recognize changes in their behaviour or emotions because of its gradual manifestation and the distancing strategies they are using.

Research about the causes, contexts, and consequences of compassion fatigue continue to develop, with greater recognition that more investment is needed in developing sociological and cultural understandings of the phenomena. Evidence is equivocal about what predisposes some nurses to compassion fatigue: for example, the balance between environmental factors or individual personality traits (such as high emotional sensitivity) or personal history (such as a personal history of trauma) (Turgoose and Maddox 2017). Similarly, the mechanisms by which compassion fatigue occurs are debated. Some theorists emphasize that it is the repeated and intense nature of suffering that nurses 'witness' that contributes to their emotional exhaustion (Salmond et al. 2019). Implicit in this explanation is that compassion fatigue reflects a state of depletion in a carer's compassion reserves. However, more recent studies have identified that experienced nurses are least likely to experience compassion fatigue, suggesting that compassion does not exist in a finite quantity ready to be depleted over the professional life course (Sinclair et al. 2017). This finding troubles the idea that caring inevitably 'costs' and that there is a linear relationship between caring and compassion fatigue (Coetzee and Laschinger 2018). Furthermore, there is limited research indicating a clear association between seemingly 'high risk' or 'emotionally intensive' nursing settings and higher rates of compassion fatigue. For example, nurses working in critical care and oncology—who potentially witness 'more' trauma and are engaging in consistently demanding emotional work—are not found to experience compassion fatigue more often than nurses who work in other, seemingly less 'traumatic', settings (Sinclair et al. 2017). This suggests that factors such as organizational culture and personal factors (e.g. ways of coping, access to support) may play a more important role in determining if and how nurses experience compassion fatigue, rather than the nature of their work per se.

Compassion fatigue is a complex personal, social, and professional phenomenon. Awareness of this has helped to shift the conceptualization of compassion fatigue from a problem primarily of individual nurses and their emotional or moral character to the recognition that addressing compassion fatigue will require healthcare organizations to take on a greater role. For example, this can be achieved by attending to programmes of training, staffing levels, management structures, and workplace cultures so that they better enable compassionate and sustainable practice (Salmond et al. 2019). Ledoux (2015) suggests that understanding why some nurses experience 'compassion satisfaction', 'compassionate resilience', and high levels of empathic ability throughout their working lives may also hold valuable insights about how to prevent compassionate fatigue.

> **Reflection Point: Caring for Jerome**
> Reflecting on Jerome's situation and the information above about compassion fatigue and moral distress, consider the following questions:
>
> - What evidence is there that members of the team caring for Jerome are experiencing (1) compassion fatigue and/or (2) moral distress?
> - Focus on the concept that you find most applicable. What are the possible effects on (1) individual members of the care team? (2) Jerome?
> - Think about what it would be like to work in this team. What might be the impact (in the short and longer term) of colleagues having different emotional and ethical responses to Jerome's situation? What support might the team need to recognize and potentially address these differences?

Vicarious Trauma

The theory of vicarious trauma is grounded in counselling practice, in which trauma is primarily experienced through inviting and listening to clients' accounts; however, a growing number of 'helping' professions have found the concept of vicarious trauma helpful in exploring the impact of working in different trauma-related situations. For nurses, the concept has helped to surface the enduring impact of having their physical or emotional safety compromised in the course of traumatic and risk-laden work.

Vicarious trauma is experienced by therapists or caregivers who exhibit signs of trauma as a direct result of their work with clients/patients who are traumatized. This does not mean that any professional working with a victim of trauma will themselves be traumatized: trauma is not an infectious disease that can be passed on through proximity to other people's trauma. Rather, McCann and Pearlman (1990)—two therapists who developed the concept—characterize vicarious trauma as occurring when (1) therapists commit to empathic engagement and exposure to graphic and traumatizing material during the therapeutic process, (2) the therapist is exposed to human cruelty, and (3) there is re-enactment of trauma within the therapy process. Vicarious trauma, therefore, involves intensive and emotionally challenging engagement with clients/patients. The work is usually prolonged and repetitive and, in this way, is different from the conditions that may give rise to compassion fatigue and burnout. Furthermore, vicarious trauma is often used interchangeably with 'secondary trauma', and for some researchers and theorists, there is little to differentiate the two conditions. However, vicarious trauma tends to be associated with a therapist/caregiver who becomes traumatized through repeated encounters with distressing or emotionally challenging accounts/events. In contrast, secondary trauma can be 'acute' (i.e. immediate) and does not necessitate the same relational conditions between the therapist/professional and their client/patient (Newell and MacNeil 2010).

Professionals affected by vicarious trauma are likely to experience profound emotional exhaustion and heightened emotional dysregulation in a similar way to compassion fatigue or burnout. Physical and somatic symptoms include but are not limited to sleep disturbance and insomnia, difficulty regulating perspiration, predisposition to chronic illness and change in appetite (Isobel and Thomas 2022). Psychological symptoms may encompass feelings of anxiety and/or depression and lowered self-esteem. Unlike compassion fatigue and burnout, vicarious trauma is also associated with a more fundamental re-ordering of a person's cognitive schema or 'worldview', which has attendant effects on a person's psychological health and social relationships. That is, the professional's sense of self, ability to trust, sense of safety, and the importance they attach to intimate relationships may alter because of their indirect exposure to trauma (Pearlman and Saakvitne 1995). In this way, vicarious trauma overlaps in some ways with post-traumatic stress disorder (PTSD), although people working in a professional capacity tend to experience trauma in a less severe or enduring way than the person/people who suffered a primary trauma (Tabor 2011).

A recent systematic literature review of the impact of traumatic births on healthcare providers characterized these professionals as the 'second victims' of traumatic births (Shorey and Wong 2021). Reviewed studies indicated that healthcare professionals had intense emotional responses during and immediately after the traumatic birth, with many professionals experiencing intrusive feelings of guilt and blame. This led to some professionals choosing to leave the profession, while others noticed changes in their intimate personal relationships, for example, because they felt more protective of loved ones or fearful about what might happen to them (Shorey and Wong 2021). Vicarious trauma has also helped to make visible the effects of forensic nurses working with victims of sexual assault. A study by Wies and Coy (2013) found that a majority of participating nurses exhibited clinical or sub-clinical signs of vicarious trauma. The researchers argue that we need to improve the identification of vicarious trauma among nurses because of the lasting and profound impacts on individuals and, in turn, the likelihood that this will negatively affect the care they can provide. Wies and Coy (2013) also argue that it is important to recognize that the stigmatized nature of sexual violence contributed to the nurses' indirect trauma because there were few opportunities to make sense of or challenge the gendered violence they witnessed and responded to on a daily basis.

Vicarious trauma offers us a theoretical framework to understand how some nurses become traumatized in the course of their work. In this respect, it is perhaps unsurprising that some of the strategies proposed to combat vicarious trauma share common ground with actions to address compassion fatigue. At the individual level, for example, evidence suggests that nurses who engage in self-care strategies, who have a robust support network, and who feel comfortable articulating their feelings are less likely to experience vicarious trauma (Isobel and Thomas 2022). It is also thought that professionals who have experienced personal trauma are more likely to be re-traumatized through certain types of therapeutic or caring work (Adams and Riggs 2008). It is, therefore, recommended that nurses have training and education around vicarious trauma so they can be better attuned to their own strengths and sensitivities. This awareness may, in turn, help nurses to make informed decisions about the type of nursing work they engage in, as well as being more alert to the needs of colleagues. Given the exacting impacts of vicarious trauma, it is important to note that some professionals develop new abilities and resources when working in challenging contexts, which enable them to recover from the initial effects of indirect trauma and, often, to continue nursing and caring in the context of trauma (Beck et al. 2017). At an organizational level, the provision of regular and good quality supervision, the guarantee of realistic workloads, and the fostering of a culture of openness and transparency may also help nurses recognize and process the complex emotions often generated when working in contexts of trauma (Shorey and Wong 2021).

We now present our second case study: Frances. When reading about Frances' situation, consider how the concepts of vicarious trauma and compassion fatigue might be relevant.

Case Study Two: Frances

Frances was brought into the ED after she was sexually and physically assaulted. The ED physician with extensive experience states that Frances' facial fractures were the worst that he had seen in his entire career. Frances is admitted to the trauma unit, and for the first 48 h, she barely moves. The nursing team—who have experience providing care to patients who have been in motor vehicle accidents or life-altering injuries such as spinal cord injuries—are at a loss at how best to care for Frances. They want to provide personal care for Frances so that she can have her cuts and bruises cleaned, but they do not want to exacerbate her trauma experience by providing intimate care that she is not ready for. The physicians prescribe post-exposure prophylaxis because they know nothing about the perpetrator of the assault. After 48 h, Frances starts screaming and crying, and then exhausting herself, she falls into a deep sleep. The nursing team tried their best to provide Frances with medication by crushing it into yoghurt and into high-calorie milkshakes in the hope that they can provide her with some nutrition. The healthcare team are inexperienced with sexual assault, so they seek the input of the sexual assault nurse examiner, Gina, who comes to assess Frances. Gina is highly experienced in her role, and she comments to the nursing team her shock and horror regarding the extent of Frances' injuries. After examining Frances, Gina talks to the nursing team about ways in which they could enhance their practice to accommodate Frances' needs. While some of the members of the nursing team feel relieved to be provided with this additional education, others feel guilty about the fact they felt so ill-equipped to care for Frances effectively.

(continued)

Frances' husband, Anthony, has been at her bedside since she was transferred from the ED. Anthony tries to assist the nursing team by encouraging Frances to eat, drink, and take her medications. It is clear that he feels lost and powerless to help Frances, as she is barely able to speak.

The charge nurse assigns Gemma to care for Frances on the fifth day of Frances' hospitalization. Gemma had been dreading being assigned to care for Frances. Gemma was sexually assaulted a few years previously, and she did not want to tell her colleagues, so rather than request a different assignment, she cares for Frances. After her shift, Gemma asks her colleagues if they want to grab a drink; she wants to try to decompress and try to forget the day. When she gets home, she finds she is unable to sleep and lays in bed, dreading her next shift.

Reflection Point: Caring for Frances
Reflecting on Frances's situation and thinking about what you have read in the section above on the impact of caring in the context of trauma, consider the following questions:

- Why might Gemma's recent experience of sexual assault affect how she feels about caring for Frances? How could the concept of vicarious trauma help to understand her experiences?
- Identify some of the ways that Anthony might be affected by Frances's experience of serious sexual assault and 'bearing witness' to her trauma in the immediate aftermath of the assault. What might be the strengths and limitations of using the concepts of vicarious trauma in a family/intimate relationships situation?

Family Caregivers

Across the globe, it is within 'informal' systems and relationships that most care takes place. Families are the single largest group of caregivers for older people, with elder spouses and adult children being the family members most likely to take on the role of caregiver (Pinquart and Sörensen 2011). While family and intimate relationships can be a source of trauma, repairing these relationships—or forging new ones—is often an integral part of growth and development across the human life course. Nevertheless, efforts to qualify, quantify, and theorize the impact of family or kinship caring has received comparably less attention than the impact on professional or 'formal' carers, such as nurses (Lynch and Lobo 2012). Furthermore, until recently, there has been very limited recognition of the experiences of family caregivers in the context of trauma. What research and practice that does exist tends to focus on the experience of foster carers (who in some senses are both 'expert' carers as well as family members) and adoptive parents looking after a child who is known to have experienced trauma or abuse. In the following section, we will explore two ways of thinking about the impact of caring and how these understandings may shape the way we understand caring in the context of trauma.

Counting the 'Cost' of Caring

Over the past three decades, there has been increased awareness of the considerable effects that caring can have on people's physical and mental health. This is sometimes referred to as the 'caregiver burden' or 'caregiver stress' theory, and it shares conceptual ground with the concept of compassion fatigue and burnout. In comparison to the general population, effects of caring include the following: increased rates of poor mobility and signs of general ageing, high rates of stress, anxiety and depression-related symptoms, and increased rates of isolation and loneliness (Carmichael and Ercolani 2016). Perhaps unsurprisingly, the degree to which family carers are 'at risk' of these negative outcomes is related to the nature and duration of care that they undertake and their social and economic circumstances. That is, people who care for longer periods or engage in different 'types' of care (e.g. meeting personal care needs, providing emotional or psychological support, practical help, etc.) are more likely to experience negative effects (Aoun et al. 2013; Ge and Mordiffi 2017). It is also the case that individuals respond differently to caring situations: personality factors play a role; however, the degree to which we anticipate (and are socialized) to expect to take on caring roles, combined with the quality and nature of our past relationships with a family member, all combine to affect how we experience caring (Chiao et al. 2015).

Recognizing the 'cost' of caring can make visible the hidden impact of caring. It can also help to identify and develop the support and help for family carers: for example, training and education programmes, investment in respite care, and exploration of therapeutic or psycho-social support programmes (Miko et al. 2022; Rolbiecki et al. 2020). Recognizing the impact of caring can also help to raise awareness of the social and economic contribution that family carers make and their integral role in enabling 'formal' health and social care systems to operate, often with a huge cost saving to government and/or private providers. For some campaigning groups, demonstrating the cost of caring helps to make the case for an increased distribution of resources (e.g. for improved services) and helps to give family caring parity of esteem with professional carers.

Nevertheless, critics argue that much of the research and narrative around the 'caregiver burden' is unduly pessimistic and does not reflect the complexity and diversity of most people's experiences of caring (Purkis and Ceci 2015). Suggesting that family caring is different from professional caring in the sense only that family carers are not 'trained' (implying that they lack skills and knowledge) and that it is more intensive (i.e. because family carers often carry out more hours of care) potentially fails to acknowledge the ethical and social contexts in which people take on and inhabit caring roles. It also tends to minimize 'non-visible' dimensions of caring dynamics, such as the expenditure of emotional labour, particularly when carried out on a regular or long-term basis (Larkin et al. 2019). This, in turn, affects how we identify and respond to caring in the context of trauma.

Caring for Family Members: Ethics of Care Perspective

There is a small but growing body of research that conceptualizes giving and receiving care as primarily relational and emotional experiences that people engage in throughout their lives (for example Barnes 2012; Kittay 2011). This ethics of care perspective challenges the framing of care as a prescribed set of tasks predicated by an individual's physical or psychological health needs and argues that family care needs to be understood within a broader context. If we examine the broader context, then we see how 'private' and 'personal' spaces are significantly shaped by the (unequal) distribution of social and political resources family (Kittay 2009). The low social and economic value placed on formal and family care practices reflects latent assumptions that caring is a 'natural' exercise: an expression of common humanity or empathy, and one that women are socially conditioned to value and to accept in their personal and professional lives (Lynch 2007). Instead, ethics of care scholars argue that caring is a multi-dimensional, dynamic process that is foregrounded in inter-dependent and reciprocal relationships that are often based on identities and commitments forged across the life course (Fine and Glendinning 2005; Forbat 2005).

From this perspective, the experience of caring for a family member or partner is not primarily understood as a 'burden' or 'cost' to be shouldered. Instead, caring can present an opportunity to negotiate new relationships and intimacies based on a mutual understanding of changing roles and needs (Larkin et al. 2019). This can lead to a new or renewed sense of emotional closeness between family members. This may come about as the result of negotiated routines, spaces, and decisions as necessitated by a person's changing health needs. Furthermore, although ethics of care scholars challenge the idea that caring is a transactional process, there is recognition that many carers report a sense of 'giving back' and of fulfilling ethical and relational duties in caring for a partner or family member who has supported them at another point in life (Barnes 2012). For example, for adult children caring for a parent in old age or for adults in a long-term partnership. For families where relationships have not always been harmonious, there is evidence to suggest that some people experience caring roles as a chance to repair and recalibrate. For example, changing patterns of dependency between family members shift the balance of power and/or control within relationships, leading to new roles and identities. Caring relationships can also offer a chance to demonstrate commitment and, for some people, to offer atonement or forgiveness for things that have happened in the past (Band-Winterstein and Eisikovits 2014).

These dynamics are particularly powerful for families affected by trauma. Trauma can affect families in complex and distinct ways, and there is often no one single cause of familial trauma, even when there is collective suffering. It is also the case that for some families, their primary trauma is rooted in their experiences of receiving inconsistent or damaging care from other family members. This offers insights into why, for some families, caring in the context of trauma may be particularly challenging (Blood and Guthrie 2018; Lim and Fathi 2020). Research indicates that people who have had difficult relationships with family members in the past are likely to find it more emotionally difficult caring for them in later life, and this, in turn, may lead to carers employing coping mechanisms that include withdrawal and distancing strategies (and, less frequently, neglectful or abusive practices) that result in their family members' needs not being met (Isham et al. 2019). Alternatively, some people may find it hard to manage their intense emotions, and this may result in difficulties empathizing with or anticipating another person's needs and may result, in extreme situations, in verbal or physical violence (Reder and Duncan 2001). It is, therefore, not realistic or desirable for everyone to give or receive care from their family members (or partners), particularly when there is a history of unresolved trauma. Furthermore, it is important to recognize that family trauma is often 'hidden' and that proactive, empathic exploration is often required to help families reach informed decisions about the most appropriate ways to care and support one another as their needs change.

> **Reflection on Frances and Anthony at Home**
> - Thinking about the nurses' interactions with Anthony in the hospital, how might health professionals contribute to expectations around caring roles in families? How does a feminist ethics of care perspective help us to understand the way care is understood and 'performed'?
> - Frances and Anthony have experienced considerable changes in their roles and their circumstances that began with Frances' experience of sexual assault. What are the challenges they are facing? What opportunities might there be for positive change or personal/relational growth?

> **Frances: Returning Home**
> On the third night of Frances' admission, Anthony decided to go home for a shower and to sleep properly but the nurses had seemed so shocked that after that he stayed on a cot in her room for the rest of her week-long hospital stay. When he had returned, the nurses had helped him to feel more comfortable by bringing him blankets and cups of tea, and they reassured him how important it was that Frances had someone she loved and trusted nearby.

(continued)

> Back at home, Anthony and Frances are finding it difficult to adjust and to process what has happened. Anthony has had to return to work (with Frances taking time off, they are relying on Anthony's salary to pay the bills), leaving Frances alone throughout the day. Frances begs him to come home as she feels frightened being alone and is experiencing flashbacks and anxiety attacks. Frances does not want to tell her parents or sister about what has happened, in part because she feels ashamed but also because she does not know how they will respond: they have always been difficult to 'read' and never been close. What support would they be now? In the month since returning from the hospital, Frances is starting to feel increasingly isolated, and her mental health is worsening. Frances feels frustrated and upset that Anthony is not helping her more; Anthony feels that no matter what he does, it is never enough, and he no longer knows if he is helping Frances.

Summary

This chapter has provided an introduction to the impact of trauma on formal and family caregivers through the lens of care ethics and feminist ethics. In the first section, there is an introduction to care ethics, feminist ethics, and common ethical theories that are important within healthcare. These theories provide the grounding from which the ethical obligations and responsibilities of formal and family caregivers are explored, including considerations of ways in which one's responsibilities might come into conflict.

The concepts of moral distress, compassion fatigue, and vicarious trauma are described, including controversies and debates about how these concepts are appropriately understood and responded to in clinical practice. Through the case study of Jerome, the sub-categories of moral distress are explored from the perspectives of different members of the healthcare team. In the second case study of Frances, the reader is encouraged to consider the concepts of compassion fatigue and vicarious trauma and the ways in which these occur for both formal and family caregivers.

Finally, this chapter explored how experiences of caring for family members remain less visible and well-understood in comparison to caring in professional settings. This matters when, across the globe, so much of caring 'work' is carried out in domestic spaces and within familial and kinship relationships. This chapter discussed how caring can be understood as exerting a 'cost'—e.g. because of its impact on people's physical and mental health or disruption to their employment. Feminist ethics of care scholars suggest that caring can also be understood primarily in ethical and relational terms and that this lens better helps us understand the emotional and social context of caring, as well as its gendered and cultural nature. We suggest that these perspectives provide valuable ways of understanding caring in the context of trauma for families. They also alert us to the additional challenges that trauma is likely to create for care relationships within families across the life course.

This chapter aimed to introduce you, the reader, to research and theory that considers the nature and impact of caring practices, with a focus on the ethical, emotional, and social impacts of caring in distressing or difficult situations. The case studies were intended as exercises to consider the link between this theory and research, and nursing and family care 'in practice'. This chapter is intended to help you reflect—at different points in your career—on the value as well as the impact that caring has had on you in your personal and professional life. It may also inform your decisions about what kind of setting you practice in, how you work with colleagues, and, critically, how you support and work in partnership with families (see Table 6.2 for recent developments and description of concepts).

Table 6.2 Concepts and recent controversy

Description of concept/phenomenon	Recent significant research and controversy
Burnout: Burnout is a 'psychological syndrome of emotional exhaustion, depersonalization, and reduced personal accomplishment that can occur among individuals who work with other people in some capacity' (Maslach et al. 1997), p. 192)	Rushton et al. (2015) explored several factors believed to affect the retention and turnover of nursing personnel in 'high-intensity settings': burnout, moral distress, stress, resilience, meaning, and hope. Both moral distress and resilience were statistically significantly correlated to all three aspects of burnout (emotional exhaustion, depersonalization, personal accomplishment), indicating that where moral distress scored highly, so did burnout, while greater resilience was correlated with lower scores. The authors concluded that moral distress predicted burnout, whereas greater resilience mitigated it (Rushton et al. 2015) Dall'Ora et al. (2020) suggest that more research needs to be conducted to understand the associations between burnout and nurse turnover
Compassion fatigue: 'An acute onset of physical and emotional responses that culminate in a decrease in compassionate feelings towards others because of an individual's occupation' (Sinclair et al. 2017, p. 10)	The need to develop an empirical and theoretical understanding of compassion fatigue specific to the context of nursing, and the way in which it differs from 'empathy' and 'sympathy.' Recently, some scholars have highlighted the potential dangers of empathy as leading to burnout and exhaustion. Bloom (2017) suggests that empathy can also derail moral decision-making because it heightens emotions and exacerbates the potential for bias
Emotional labour: To care for patients, nurses may be required to manage or suppress feelings of disgust, fear, or horror at the situations they encounter. This act of regulating one's emotions to fulfil the expectations of a job is called 'emotional labor' (Hochschild 2012)	Emotional labour has been taken up by a number of nurse researchers and theorists and is widely considered to be a valuable way of conceptualizing the emotional, affective, and (often) gendered dimensions of the nursing role (Gray 2010)

(continued)

Table 6.2 (continued)

Description of concept/phenomenon	Recent significant research and controversy
Moral injury: Shay (2014) states that moral injury occurs when there is (i) a betrayal of what is right, (ii) in a high stakes situation, (iii) by someone who holds legitimate authority	Following the COVID-19 pandemic, there has been increased use of the term 'moral injury' in healthcare settings. However, the empirical evidence is still limited, and it is often not clear what the differences are between 'moral distress', 'burnout', and 'moral injury'. There is a need for more conceptual work to understand the differences between moral distress and moral injury as experienced by healthcare workers
Vicarious trauma: Drawing on the work of McCann & Pearlmann (1990), Baird and Kracen (2006) characterize vicarious traumatization as follows: 'harmful changes that occur in professionals' views of themselves, others, and the world as a result of exposure to graphic and/or traumatic material. Vicarious trauma can be seen as a normal response to ongoing challenges to a helper's beliefs and values but can result in decreased motivation, efficacy, and empathy'	Much of the research base is inter-disciplinary, and there is a need for nursing-specific empirical and conceptual work to 'test' the theory and adapt it to the nursing context. Most research and theory focus on defining and explaining the problem. Future work could focus more on proposed prevention and intervention strategies. There remains conceptual confusion between vicarious trauma, compassion fatigue, and burnout. It is unclear whether this makes any difference in practice.

Discussion Questions

1. What are three ethical considerations that are significant for nurses when caring for patients who have experienced trauma?
2. Describe moral distress, compassion fatigue, and vicarious trauma and discuss how these might impact formal caregivers.
3. Discuss the ways in which trauma can impact family caregivers and the ways in which nurses might support family caregivers (Box 6.4).

Box 6.3: Reflection Box

Use the reflective questions in this box as an exercise to explore your motivations to work as a nurse, and/or in a trauma setting, and to consider the supports you may need in your career as a nurse:

1. What motivated you to train as a nurse?
2. If you are considering working in a trauma setting, what interests you about that specialty?
3. What do you think you need with regard to support and resources to be successful working in a trauma setting?
4. What are some of the strengths that you bring to your work, and specifically to a trauma setting?

> **Box 6.4: List of Resources**
> **American Association of Critical-Care Nurses**
> Moral distress: https://www.aacn.org/clinical-resources/moral-distress
>
> **American Nurses Association**
> Healthy Nurse, Healthy Nation Campaign: https://www.healthynursehealthynation.org/?__hstc=53609399.35f3bd92022a157931cd6666d01c3f95.1648942003031.1649940122980.1649963550504.3&__hssc=53609399.2.1649963550504&__hsfp=3385294858
>
> **British Medical Association**
> Vicarious Trauma: https://www.bma.org.uk/advice-and-support/your-wellbeing/vicarious-trauma/vicarious-trauma-signs-and-strategies-for-coping#:~:text=Vicarious%20trauma%20is%20a%20process,doctors%20and%20other%20health%20professionals
>
> **Pan American Health Organization**
> Mental health in the workplace: https://www.paho.org/en/file/49121/download?token=7NxfBnVS
>
> **United Nations**
> Formal and Informal Caregivers Policy Brief: https://unece.org/DAM/pau/age/Policy_briefs/ECE_WG1_31.pdf
>
> **World Health Organization**
> Burnout: https://www.who.int/tools/occupational-hazards-in-health-sector/occup-stress-burnout-fatigue
>
> **WHO Global Plan of Action on Workers' Health (2008–2017):** https://www.who.int/publications/i/item/WHO-FWC-PHE-2013-01

References

Adams SA, Riggs SA (2008) An exploratory study of vicarious trauma among therapist trainees. Train Educ Prof Psychol 2(1):26–34. https://doi.org/10.1037/1931-3918.2.1.26

American Nurses Association, ANA (2025) Code of Ethics for Nurses. https://codeofethics.ana.org/home

Amos VK, Epstein E (2022) Moral distress interventions: an integrative literature review. Nurs Ethics 29(3):582–607. https://doi.org/10.1177/09697330211035489

Anscombe GEM (1958) Modern moral philosophy. Philosophy 33(124):1–19. https://doi.org/10.1017/S0031819100037943

Aoun SM, Bentley B, Funk L, Toye C, Grande G, Stajduhar KJ (2013) A 10-year literature review of family caregiving for motor neurone disease: moving from caregiver burden studies to palliative care interventions. Palliat Med 27(5):437–446. https://doi.org/10.1177/0269216312455729

Baird K, Kracen AC (2006) Vicarious traumatization and secondary traumatic stress: a research synthesis. Couns Psychol Q 19(2):181–188. https://doi.org/10.1080/09515070600811899

Band-Winterstein T, Eisikovits Z (2014) Intimate violence across the lifespan: interpersonal, familial, and cross-generational perspectives. Springer Science + Business Media. https://doi.org/10.1007/978-1-4939-1354-1

Barnes M (2012) Care in everyday life: an ethic of care in practice. Policy Press

Beauchamp TL, Childress JF (2013) Principles of biomedical ethics, 7th edn. Oxford University Press

Beauchamp TL, Childress JF (2015) Principles of biomedical ethics (7th edition). Oxford University Press.

Beck CT, Rivera J, Gable RK (2017) A mixed-methods study of vicarious posttraumatic growth in certified nurse-midwives. J Midwifery Womens Health 62(1):80–87. https://doi.org/10.1111/jmwh.12523

Blood I, Guthrie L (2018) Supporting older people using attachment-informed and strengths-based approaches. Jessica Kingsley Publishing. https://academic.oup.com/bjsw/article-abstract/49/6/1690/5303233

Bloom P (2017) Empathy and its discontents. Trends Cogn Sci 21(1):24–31. https://doi.org/10.1016/j.tics.2016.11.004

Campbell SM, Ulrich CM, Grady C (2016) A broader understanding of moral distress. Am J Bioeth: AJOB 16(12):2–9. https://doi.org/10.1080/15265161.2016.1239782

Card C (1990) Caring and evil. Hypatia 5(1):101–108. https://doi.org/10.1111/j.1527-2001.1990.tb00393.x

Carmichael F, Ercolani MG (2016) Unpaid caregiving and paid work over life-courses: different pathways, diverging outcomes. Soc Sci Med 1982(156):1–11. https://doi.org/10.1016/j.socscimed.2016.03.020

Chiao C-Y, Wu H-S, Hsiao C-Y (2015) Caregiver burden for informal caregivers of patients with dementia: A systematic review. Int Nurs Rev 62(3):340–350. https://doi.org/10.1111/inr.12194

Coetzee SK, Laschinger HKS (2018) Toward a comprehensive, theoretical model of compassion fatigue: an integrative literature review. Nurs Health Sci 20(1):4–15. https://doi.org/10.1111/nhs.12387

Dall'Ora C, Ball J, Reinius M, Griffiths P (2020) Burnout in nursing: a theoretical review. Hum Resour Health 18(1):41. https://doi.org/10.1186/s12960-020-00469-9

Epstein EG, Hurst AR, Mahanes D, Marshall MF, Hamric AB (2016) Is Broader Better? Am J Bioeth: AJOB 16(12):15–17. https://doi.org/10.1080/15265161.2016.1242669

Figley CR (2013) Compassion fatigue: coping with secondary traumatic stress disorder in those who treat the traumatized. Routledge. https://www.routledge.com/Compassion-Fatigue-Coping-With-Secondary-Traumatic-Stress-Disorder-In-Those/Figley/p/book/9781138884441

Fine M, Glendinning C (2005) Dependence, independence or inter-dependence? Revisiting the concepts of 'care' and 'dependency'. Ageing Soc 25(4):601–621. https://doi.org/10.1017/S0144686X05003600

Forbat L (2005) Talking about care: two sides to the story. Policy Press

Fourie C (2015) Moral distress and moral conflict in clinical ethics. Bioethics 29(2):91–97. https://doi.org/10.1111/bioe.12064

Fowler MD (2016) Nursing's code of ethics, social ethics, and social policy. Hast Cent Rep 46(Suppl 1):S9–S12. https://doi.org/10.1002/hast.624

Frankena WK (1983) Moral-point-of-view theories. In: Ethical theory in the last quarter of the twentieth century. Bowie NE (ed) Indianapolis: Hackett Publishing Company.

Fry ST (1989) The role of caring in a theory of nursing ethics. Hypatia 4(2):88–103

Fry ST, Johnstone M-J (2002) Ethics in nursing practice, 2nd edn. Blackwell

Gadow SA (1985) Nurse and patient: the caring relationship. In: Bishop AH, Scudder JR (eds) Caring, curing, coping: nurse, physician, patient relationships. University of Alabama Press, University, AL, pp. 31–43

Ge L, Mordiffi SZ (2017) Factors associated with higher caregiver burden among family caregivers of elderly cancer patients: A systematic review. Cancer Nurs 40(6):471–478. https://doi.org/10.1097/NCC.0000000000000445

Gilligan C (1982) In a different voice: psychological theory and women's development. Harvard University Press

Gotlib A (2022) Feminist ethics and narrative ethics [Online]. The Internet Encyclopaedia of Philosophy. http://www.iep.utm.edu/fem-e-n/

Gowans CW (1987) The debate on moral dilemmas. In: Moral dilemmas. Oxford University Press

Gray B (2010) Emotional labour, gender and professional stereotypes of emotional and physical contact, and personal perspectives on the emotional labour of nursing. J Gend Stud 19(4):349–360. https://doi.org/10.1080/09589236.2010.514207

Hochschild AR (2012) The managed heart: commercialization of human feeling, updated with a new preface, 3rd edn. University of California Press

ICN, I. C. of N (2021) The ICN code of ethics for nurses. https://www.icn.ch/system/files/2021-10/ICN_Code-of-Ethics_EN_Web_0.pdf

Imbulana DI, Davis PG, Prentice TM (2021) Interventions to reduce moral distress in clinicians working in intensive care: a systematic review. Intensive Crit Care Nurs 66:103092. https://doi.org/10.1016/j.iccn.2021.103092

Isham L, Hewison A, Bradbury-Jones C (2019) When older people are violent or abusive toward their family caregiver: a review of mixed-methods research. Trauma Violence Abuse 20(5):626–637. https://doi.org/10.1177/1524838017726425

Isobel S, Thomas M (2022) Vicarious trauma and nursing: an integrative review. Int J Ment Health Nurs 31(2):247–259. https://doi.org/10.1111/inm.12953

Jaggar AM (1991) Feminist ethics: projects, problems, propsects. In: Card, C. (ed.) Feminist Ethics. Lawrence: University Press of Kansas.

Jaggar AM (2001) Encyclopedia of ethics. In: Becker LC, Becker CB (eds) Encyclopedia of ethics. Routledge

Jameton A (1984) Nursing practice: the ethical issue. Prentice Hall

Johnstone M-J (2009) Bioethics: a nursing perspective, 5th edn. Elsevier. https://www.elsevier.com/books/bioethics/johnstone/978-0-7295-4322-4

Kelly L, Runge J, Spencer C (2015) Predictors of compassion fatigue and compassion satisfaction in acute care nurses. J Nurs Scholarship 47(6):522–528. https://doi.org/10.1111/jnu.12162

Kittay EF (2009) The personal is philosophical is political: a philosopher and mother of a cognitively disabled person sends notes from the battlefield. Metaphilosophy 40(3–4):606. https://onlinelibrary.wiley.com/doi/full/10.1111/j.1467-9973.2009.01600.x

Kittay EF (2011) The ethics of care, dependence, and disability. Ratio Juris 24(1):49–58

Kohlberg L (1981) The philosophy of moral development: moral stages and the idea of justice. Harber & Row

Kohlen H (2020) Hospital ethics committees and the dismissal of nursing ethical concerns: A feminist perspective. In: Kohlen H, McCarthy J (eds) Nursing ethics: feminist perspectives. Springer

Kok N, Van Gurp J, van der Hoeven JG, Fuchs M, Hoedemaekers C, Zegers M (2021) Complex interplay between moral distress and other risk factors of burnout in ICU professionals: findings from a cross-sectional survey study. BMJ Qual Saf 32:225. https://doi.org/10.1136/bmjqs-2020-012239

Korsgaard CM (1997) Introduction. In: Ameriks C, Clarke DM (eds) Groundwork of the metaphysics of morals. Cambridge University Press

Kuhse H (1997) Caring: nurses, women and ethics. Blackwell Publishers Ltd

Larkin M, Henwood M, Milne A (2019) Carer-related research and knowledge: findings from a scoping review. Health Soc Care Community 27(1):55–67. https://doi.org/10.1111/hsc.12586

Ledoux K (2015) Understanding compassion fatigue: understanding compassion. J Adv Nurs 71(9):2041–2050. https://doi.org/10.1111/jan.12686

Lim HJ, Fathi M (2020) Parenting and care in adulthood: an intersectional framework for support. In: Human growth and development in adults. Policy Press. https://policy.bristoluniversitypress.co.uk/human-growth-and-development-in-adults

Lynch K (2007) Love labour as a distinct and non-Commodifiable form of care labour. Sociol Rev 55(3):550. https://doi.org/10.1111/j.1467-954X.2007.00714.x

Lynch SH, Lobo ML (2012) Compassion fatigue in family caregivers: a Wilsonian concept analysis. J Adv Nurs 68(9):2125–2134. https://doi.org/10.1111/j.1365-2648.2012.05985.x

MacIntyre A (1981) From Homer to Benjamin Franklin: the nature of the virtues. Hast Cent Rep 11(2):27–34

Maslach C, Jackson SE, Leiter MP (1997) Maslach burnout inventory: third edition. In: Evaluating stress: a book of resources. Scarecrow Education, pp 191–218

McCann IL, Pearlman LA (1990) Vicarious traumatization: a framework for understanding the psychological effects of working with victims. J Trauma Stress 3(1):131–149. https://doi.org/10.1007/BF00975140

McCarthy J (2006) A pluralist view of nursing ethics. Nurs Philos 7(3):157–164. https://doi.org/10.1111/j.1466-769X.2006.00272.x

McLeod-Sordjan R (2014) Evaluating moral reasoning in nursing education. Nurs Ethics 21(4):473–483. https://doi.org/10.1177/0969733013505309

Miko AL, Berger E, Krishnamoorthy G (2022) Exploring self-care practices in foster carers: a qualitative study. J Publ Child Welfare 17:1–23. https://doi.org/10.1080/15548732.2022.2027844

Morley G, Bradbury-Jones C, Ives J (2020a) What is "moral distress" in nursing? A feminist empirical bioethics study. Nurs Ethics 27(5):1297–1314. https://doi.org/10.1177/0969733019874492

Morley G, Sese D, Rajendram P, Horsburgh CC (2020b) Addressing caregiver moral distress during the COVID-19 pandemic. Cleve Clin J Med. https://doi.org/10.3949/ccjm.87a.ccc047

Morley G, Field R, Horsburgh CC, Burchill C (2021a) Interventions to mitigate moral distress: a systematic review of the literature. Int J Nurs Stud 121:103984. https://doi.org/10.1016/j.ijnurstu.2021.103984

Morley G, Bradbury-Jones C, Ives J (2021b) Reasons to redefine moral distress: a feminist empirical bioethics analysis. Bioethics 35(1):61–71. https://doi.org/10.1111/bioe.12783

Morley G, Bradbury-Jones C, Ives J (2021c) The moral distress model: an empirically informed guide for moral distress interventions. J Clin Nurs 31:1309. https://doi.org/10.1111/jocn.15988

Morley G, Sankary LR, Horsburgh CC (2022) Mitigating moral distress through ethics consultation. Am J Bioeth: AJOB 22(4):61–63. https://doi.org/10.1080/15265161.2022.2044555

Nelson HL (1992) Against caring. J Clin Ethics 3(1):8–15; discussion 15-20

Newell JM, MacNeil GA (2010) Professional burnout, vicarious trauma, secondary traumatic stress, and compassion fatigue: a review of theoretical terms, risk factors, and preventive methods for clinicians and researchers. Best Pract Ment Health Int J 6(2):57–68

NMC, T. N. and M. C (2015) The code: professional standards of practice and behaviour for nurses, midwives and nursing associates. https://www.nmc.org.uk/standards/code/

Noddings N (1984) Caring: a feminine approach to ethics and education. University of California Press

Noddings N (2002) Caring, social policy, and homelessness. Theor Med Bioeth 23(6):441–454. https://doi.org/10.1023/a:1021385717732

Noddings N (2015) In: Engster E, Hamington M (eds) Care ethics and "caring" organizations in care ethics and political theory. Oxford University Press

Pearlman LA, Saakvitne KW (1995) Trauma and the therapist: countertransference and vicarious traumatization in psychotherapy with incest survivors. W W Norton & Co., p xix, 451

Peters E (2018) Compassion fatigue in nursing: a concept analysis. Nurs Forum 53(4):466–480. https://doi.org/10.1111/nuf.12274

Pinquart M, Sörensen S (2011) Spouses, adult children, and children-in-law as caregivers of older adults: A meta-analytic comparison. Psychol Aging 26(1):1–14. https://doi.org/10.1037/a0021863

Purkis ME, Ceci C (2015) Problematising care burden research. Ageing Soc 35(7):1410–1428

Reder P, Duncan S (2001) Abusive relationships, care and control conflicts and insecure attachments. Child Abuse Rev 10(6):411–427

Rolbiecki AJ, Oliver DP, Washington K, Benson JJ, Jorgensen L (2020) Preliminary results of caregiver speaks: a storytelling intervention for bereaved family caregivers. J Loss Trauma 25(5):438–453. https://doi.org/10.1080/15325024.2019.1707985

Rushton CH, Batcheller J, Schroeder K, Donohue P (2015) Burnout and resilience among nurses practicing in high-intensity settings. Am J Crit Care 24(5):412–420. https://doi.org/10.4037/ajcc2015291

Salmond E, Salmond S, Ames M, Kamienski M, Holly C (2019) Experiences of compassion fatigue in direct care nurses: a qualitative systematic review. JBI Database System Rev Implement Rep 17(5):682–753. https://doi.org/10.11124/JBISRIR-2017-003818

Shay J (2014) Moral injury. Psychoanal Psychol 32(2):182–191. https://doi.org/10.1037/a0036090

Shorey S, Wong PZE (2021) Vicarious trauma experienced by health care providers involved in traumatic childbirths: a meta-synthesis. Trauma Violence Abuse:1585. https://doi.org/10.1177/15248380211013135

Sinclair S, Raffin-Bouchal S, Venturato L, Mijovic-Kondejewski J, Smith-MacDonald L (2017) Compassion fatigue: a meta-narrative review of the healthcare literature. Int J Nurs Stud 69:9–24. https://doi.org/10.1016/j.ijnurstu.2017.01.003

Snelling PC (2016) The metaethics of nursing codes of ethics and conduct. Nurs Philos 17(4):229–249. https://doi.org/10.1111/nup.12122

Tabor PD (2011) Vicarious traumatization: concept analysis. J Forensic Nurs 7(4):203–208. https://doi.org/10.1111/j.1939-3938.2011.01115.x

Tessman L (2015) Moral failure: on the impossible demands of morality. Oxford University Press

Tigard DW (2018) Rethinking moral distress: conceptual demands for a troubling phenomenon affecting health care professionals. Med Health Care Philos 21(4):479–488. https://doi.org/10.1007/s11019-017-9819-5

Turgoose D, Maddox L (2017) Predictors of compassion fatigue in mental health professionals: a narrative review. Traumatology 23(2):172

Walker MU (2007) Moral understandings: a feminist study in ethics. Oxford University Press

Watson J (1985) Nursing human science and human care, a theory of nursing. National League for Nursing, New York

Westacott E (2022) Moral relativism [Online]. The Internet Encyclopaedia of Philosophy. https://iep.utm.edu/moral-re/#:~:text=Moral%20relativism%20is%20the%20view,uniquely%20privileged%20over%20all%20others

Wies J, Coy K (2013) Measuring violence: vicarious trauma among sexual assault nurse examiners. https://doi.org/10.17730/HUMO.72.1.X5658P957K5G7722

Wolf LA, Perhats C, Delao AM, Moon MD, Clark PR, Zavotsky KE (2016a) "It's a burden you carry": describing moral distress in emergency nursing. J Emerg Nurs 42(1):37–46. https://doi.org/10.1016/j.jen.2015.08.008

Wolf L, Ulrich CM, Grady C (2016b) Emergency nursing, Ebola, and public policy: the contributions of nursing to the public policy conversation. Hast Cent Rep 46(Suppl 1):S35–S38. https://doi.org/10.1002/hast.630

Generational Trauma 7

Eugenia Millender and Patty Wilson

Objectives
- To explore the biopsychosocial principles of generational trauma
- To describe the differences between historical, transgenerational, and intergenerational trauma
- To describe current research related to generational trauma

Introduction

Disparities contribute to trauma. A group's experience of collective traumas and social disparities based on race, ethnicity, or religion has the greatest personal impact of all traumas. Family and community members can also be affected. This can occur through direct or indirect transmission from a parent to child or multiple times over the course of an individual's, family's, or group's lifetime (Kira et al. 2019). Diverse populations developed senses of "we" that had been shaped by traumas, which reflected a collective generational trauma derived from narratives as a larger cultural transmission. In this case, traumatic memories of genocide and discrimination are shared over time by community members and/or family members as a method of sustaining their culture and unique history, leading individuals to perceive the group's experience as their own. The ability to share memories sometimes helps a person or group heal by making meaning of their trauma by connecting their

E. Millender (✉)
Florida State University, Tallahassee, FL, USA
e-mail: Emillender@fsu.edu

P. Wilson
Johns Hopkins University School of Nursing, Baltimore, MD, USA
e-mail: pwilso23@jhu.edu

past, present, and future. However, it also serves as a path for transgenerational transmission of trauma that often happens by sharing verbal stories, increasing the risk for mental disorders and the need for culturally trauma-inform care (Liehr and Smith 2020). The transmission of generational traumas can be conscious (by sharing stories), unconscious (by emotional reactions), genetic (by gene information), epigenetic (by gene function), and environmental (by the environment and its effects) (Prevention 2022). The transmission passed on to children varies by cultural background; consequently, it is essential to understand the unique risk factors that are associated with diverse groups and subgroups (Lehrner and Yehuda 2018; Özlü-Erkilic et al. 2020). Trauma can be experienced indirectly (as in transgenerational experiences), experienced directly, or witnessed (American Psychological Association 2021). Disparities in social, environmental, economic, structural, and interpersonal gradients produce experiences and emotions that induce trauma, which may manifest as one or several mental illnesses and or substance use/abuse conditions (Marmot 2018). Generational traumas may be amplified by circumstances, such as the struggle to maintain connections to one's past while living in current political and economic realities, realities that may not show deference to the historical tussles that have a real and devastating influence on the present-day well-being of certain communities and populations (Brave Heart et al. 2011).

Concepts

It is important to distinguish between the ways in which trauma is transmitted from generation to generation and the various forms of trauma that can be experienced by an individual or generation. There are two types of trauma transmission and three types of traumas that will be discussed in this chapter.

Intergenerational Trauma Transmission The transmission of trauma effects from parents (F0) to their children (F1) and grandchildren (F2) (Lehrner and Yehuda 2018; Stenz et al. 2018). It is often said that intergenerational trauma occurs from generation zero to generation two (F0 to F1 to F2)(Lehrner and Yehuda 2018). The F0 symbolizes the person who directly experienced the trauma, while the F1 and F2 symbolize the offspring of F0 with direct germ cells that trauma may have been transmitted (Yehuda et al. 2018).

Transgenerational Trauma Transmission The transmission of trauma effects between directly exposed individuals (F0) to future generations (F3 or F4 in females and F2 or F3 in males) not directly exposed to the germ's cells from F0 (Stanley and Deirdre 2019; Yehuda et al. 2018) (see Table 7.1).

Generational Trauma Type This refers to a traumatic event that is impacting individuals in many different generations post initial or direct exposure.

7 Generational Trauma

Table 7.1 Definitions

Concepts	Definition
Intergenerational trauma transmission (F0 to F1 to F2)	Trauma is directly experienced by an individual (F0) and is then passed on to their offspring (F1 and F2). See Figs. 7.1 and 7.2
Transgenerational trauma transmission (F0 to F3 or F4 females or F2 for males)	Trauma is directly experienced by an individual (F0) and passed on to future generations (F3 or F4 in females and F2 in males). See Figs. 7.1 and 7.2
Generational trauma type	Generations of trauma are transmitted in different ways from generation to generation
Cumulative trauma type	Exposure to a variety of social, psychological, and environmental stressors and traumas over a lifespan
Historical trauma type	A lifetime of victimization on a group that continuously links the past, present, and future, resulting in generational trauma

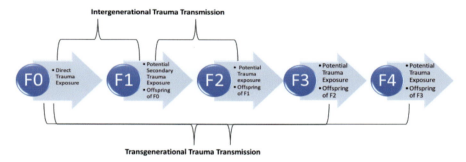

Fig. 7.1 Trauma exposure timeline

Cumulative Trauma Type This describes different types and frequency of trauma a person has been exposed to over their lifetime, while generational trauma describes the transmission of these traumas from one generation to another (see Chap. 8) (Cypress 2021; Kira et al. 2014).

Historical Trauma Type This refers to the traumas experienced by a specific cultural group that has been oppressed in a systematic manner throughout its history (Brave Heart 2003; Brave Heart et al. 2011). Some examples include the Holocaust, genocide, slavery, and forced relocation. Historical trauma can and often is passed on to other generations, resulting in transgenerational trauma. Historical trauma can be transgenerationally transmitted, as it is embedded in a lifetime of victimization and social structure consistently linking the past, the present, and the future (Stanley and Deirdre 2019).

Considering the changing face of the United States and its increasing diversity, it becomes increasingly important to understand the different forms of trauma that are experienced by all communities, as well as how this impacts future generations. It is

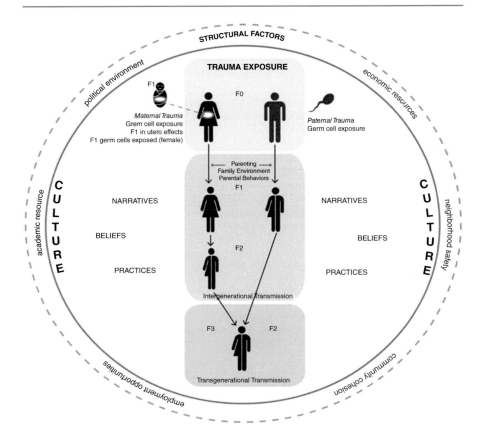

Fig. 7.2 Intergenerational transmission of biological effects of trauma

possible for individuals to be exposed to a variety of social, psychological, and environmental stressors and traumas during their lifetimes that could result in biological changes, poorer health outcomes and the transmission of diseases to future generations (Allen et al. 2014; Marmot 2005). There are many facets to trauma, which extend beyond a single traumatic event. The trauma can also be chronic, recurring, but similar to previous exposures after the exposure has ended, ongoing and repeated trauma such as discrimination, or a combination of similar and dissimilar multidimensional forms of trauma (Kira et al. 2019). As a result of adversity, high rates of psychological distress can develop, which contributes to multiple types of traumas (Gone et al. 2019). In ethnically diverse subgroups, cultural experiences are combined with complex psychosocial and environmental factors contributing to less favourable overall health outcomes (Cervantes et al. 2019). As a result of trauma, the prevalence of mental illness and substance abuse may differ depending on the type of trauma experienced (Sangalang et al. 2019). Our discussion will focus on biological, psychological, and social factors that contribute to trauma types and transmissions.

In order for trauma effects to be transmitted biologically across generations, there are multiple pathways that may be involved. The epigenetic status of maternal oocytes and paternal sperm may be affected by exposure to preconception trauma (F0); this is likely to be dependent on the individual's development, particularly in females. During embryogenesis, these effects may be conserved and manifest, resulting in the inheritance of these effects by offspring. A mother exposed to trauma during pregnancy can have an adverse effect on her foetus (F1) and the developing germline of the foetus. When the exposure occurred during pregnancy, the offspring of the foetus (F2) would have been directly exposed to the grandmother's stress (F0). Therefore, only the third generation (F3) can be considered evidence of transgenerational transmission that did not result from direct exposure. When paternal exposure occurs, F2 can be interpreted as reflecting a true transgenerational effect. Parental trauma can also be transmitted through parenting, family environment, and parental behaviour. An understanding of trauma effects and how they are transmitted is embedded within a broader biological and social-cultural context that encompasses narratives, beliefs, practices, access to resources, and the larger political environment (Lehrner and Yehuda 2018; Yehuda et al. 2018).

Biopsychosocial Framework to Exploring Generational Trauma

Assessing and exploring innovative treatment modalities for generational trauma requires utilizing holistic approaches to understand the complexity of the inheritance of traits responsible for the different transmissions and forms of trauma from one generation to another. A biopsychosocial model is flexible and adaptable, allowing for consideration of all factors that influence disease development, treatment, and transmission of disease (Engel 1977).

The biopsychosocial framework (see Fig. 7.3) is often used when discussing transgenerational trauma, giving its multidimensional and interactive approach to

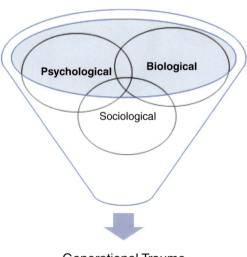

Fig. 7.3 Biopsychosocial framework for generational trauma

tackling problems by taking a holistic approach that assesses biological, psychological, and sociological factors. When completing a trauma assessment, it is important to evaluate the individual and combined effects that biological, psychological, and sociological factors have on the development and intensification of generational trauma.

Sociological Factors

Social factors are conditions that influence trauma effect transmission (see Fig. 7.4) and human behaviours by hindering day-to-day living situations when they are lacking (Wilkinson and Marmot 1998). Access to social factors differs by subcultural groups and can range from employment, education, and unsafe living conditions, which can be exacerbated by a health crisis such as COVID-19, a financial crisis such as recession, or natural disasters such as hurricanes. The severe lack of one or multiple social factors that are often rooted in systemic inequities over generations can result in stress and trauma for an individual, subcultural groups, and communities (Maxwell 2014).

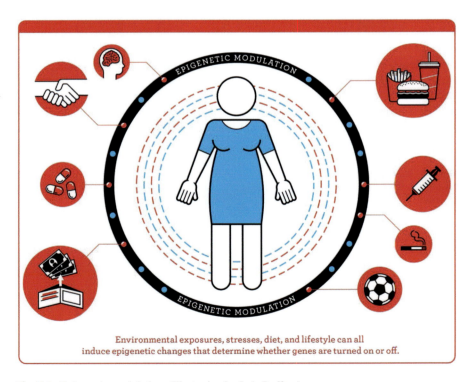

Fig. 7.4 Epigenetic modulation. (Illustration by Jude Buffum)

The impact of historical trauma is one of the most significant social and psychological factors that impact Black, Indigenous, and populations of colour. Generational trauma is in part influenced by the early experiences of a group, including factors such as genetics, early life circumstances, and lack of education that can lead to a lower socioeconomic status that later influences health status and health behaviours (Greenwood et al. 2018; Maxwell 2014). The concept of historical trauma may be defined as the accumulation of emotional and psychological wounds resulting from large-scale group traumas that are sustained over a lifetime and across generations (Brave Heart et al. 2011). Historical trauma was defined by (Kira 2001) as a systemic imprint of a complex trauma that is externally inflicted upon a particular group of individuals, which has become part of that group's everyday life. In this regard, historical trauma is susceptible to transgenerational transmission as it is rooted in a lifetime of victimization and a social structure that links the past, the present, and the future together (Millender and Lowe 2017; Power et al. 2020). Racism is one example of an early life experience that affects a generation through biological expression, which can have an impact on a gene's function as may be seen in the process of epigenetics (Taylor and Turner 2002; Taylor et al. 2016). Therefore, it is essential to address some of the traumatic past experiences so as not to silence some groups or experiences.

Exposure to toxic environmental factors such as stress, trauma, drugs, smoking, and homelessness contributes to the epigenetic transmission of trauma effects to following generations.

Psychological Factors

Behavioural and mental disorders are influenced by psychological factors, which include maintaining health and well-being, and the structure and course of their development (Lehrner and Yehuda 2018). Examples of social support include the work environment, social status, and social integration. In some cases, psychological factors may play a more significant role than biological factors; therefore, epigenetics plays a role (see Fig. 7.4).

Biological-Epigenetics Factors

Biological factors include age, gender, a genetic predisposition for trauma, neurochemistry pathology, and physiological problems. When discussing biological factors, it is important to mention the concept of epigenetics as a method of trauma transmission (Lehrner and Yehuda 2018) (see Fig. 7.4). The study of epigenetics focuses on how the environment and your behaviours contribute to changes in the way your genes function (Howard 2022).

Current Research Related to Generational Trauma

Research in the area of generational trauma has provided evidence for the complex and multifaceted effects of trauma transmission and trauma types, which can contribute to health disparities (Zannas and Chrousos 2017). Studies have also shown that trauma exposure can increase the risk for both mental and physical illness (Borsari et al. 2018; Millender and Lowe 2017). These chronic conditions are a manifestation of the trauma individuals have experienced as well as a factor in predicting and exacerbating illness. It has been demonstrated in research that providing trauma-informed assessments and care should include both a biopsychosocial model and a biosocial perspective (Howard 2022). Having a thorough understanding of symptomology associated with trauma can enhance the effectiveness of health care services. Identifying the trauma profile of culturally diverse groups or individuals will assist in identifying physical and mental disorders that they are experiencing and enable the development of trauma-informed care. A recent area of research in epigenetics is addressing the impact of parents' traumatic experiences on their offspring via intergenerational transmission (Barcelona et al. 2021). The perinatal interactional model (see Fig. 7.5) explores this phenomenon.

There are several ways in which paternal trauma (i.e. PTSD) can be transmitted to offspring: (1) in utero, which may lead to biological changes in the offspring due to parental dysregulation, and (2) after birth, as a result of parent–child interactions characterized by maladaptive parenting skills, health beliefs, and maladaptive behaviours. As a result, the child's regulatory capacity, distress level, and likelihood of developing a mental illness are affected (Lang and Gartstein 2018). Other studies are also looking at the DNA methylation changes from utero to adulthood and how these changes impact a person's risk for chronic conditions (Barcelona et al. 2021).

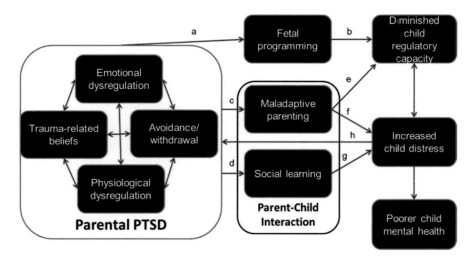

Fig. 7.5 Perinatal interactional model. (Lang and Gartstein 2018)

The field of epigenetics is still in its infancy, but studies are beginning to influence teaching curricula to include more genetics content and more genetic testing in practice.

Cases

Case Study #1

In this case, a 15-year-old female from Venezuela who received refugee status from the US Government presents with nightmares and anxiety around loud noises and adult men. She speaks Spanish only and is trying to adjust to not having her grandmother with her at the refugee shelter where she is currently housed. During the initial assessment, she reported that her grandmother raised her after her mother came to the United States when she was four. She had to stop school while in fourth grade to work to help her grandmother with the house bills. She also said she has sleeping problems because 'I can't stop thinking about my life, my past, and what is going to happen to me now'. The teenager explained that her cousins sexually abused her from age 10 to 14. She travelled alone from her home country and witnessed violence, rape, and dead bodies on her travels to the US border. She plans to reunite with her mother once she is released from the refugee shelter.

1. What topics are of priority during her trauma-focused therapy?
2. What is the role of culture during her trauma-focused therapy?
3. What is the role of social factors?

Case Study #2

Isolation can be positive and negative for many cultural groups based on their unique historical trauma experiences. Many Indigenous groups intentionally live in isolated areas such as enclaves and rural and tribal areas to sustain their language, values, and culture. When some members of this group migrated to urban places, their risk for chronic diseases increased, as well as levels of stress and trauma. An Indigenous community requested the support of health professionals to develop a culturally sensitive trauma programme due to an increase in the suicide rate and mental stress in a local Indigenous community.

1. What initial steps should one take when creating a community mental health programme for this population?
2. What are some of the potential reasons for the increase in suicide rates? Chronic health conditions?
3. How would you address the same mental health topic for different generations?

Summary

Traumatic experiences must be identified early by health professionals to prevent adverse health outcomes and the transmission of trauma to the next generation. Mental health disparities are exacerbated when complex phenomena, such as trauma, are viewed from the perspective of the clinician rather than from the viewpoint of the patient. Taking into account all forms of trauma, including cultural backgrounds, is vital for caregivers in order to contribute to a discussion regarding the inclusion of all types of trauma into a multi-global assessment that encompasses social, environmental, psychological, and biological factors. By taking a holistic and proactive approach to addressing trauma perceptions and expressions of diverse cultural groups, we will be able to construct meaningful interventions for clients, groups, and communities with diverse life experiences. Psychological factors influence behavioural and mental disorders, including their nature and course of development, as well as maintaining health and well-being. Work environment, social status, and social integration are all components of social support. Certain cases may be impacted more by psychological factors than biological factors. It is, therefore, important to take into account epigenetic factors.

Discussion Questions

1. Why are certain groups at higher risk for transgenerational trauma?
2. What are the major root causes of transgenerational trauma?
3. What are some preventative measures we can take to decrease transgenerational trauma?

References

Allen J, Balfour R, Bell R, Marmot M (2014) Social determinants of mental health. Int Rev Psychiatr (Abingdon, England) 26(4):392–407. https://doi.org/10.3109/09540261.2014.928270

American Psychological Association (2021) Trauma. https://www.apa.org/topics/trauma

Barcelona V, Montalvo-Ortiz JL, Wright ML, Nagamatsu ST, Dreisbach C, Crusto CA, Sun YV, Taylor JY (2021) DNA methylation changes in African American women with a history of preterm birth from the InterGEN study. BMC Genomic Data 22(1):30–30. https://doi.org/10.1186/s12863-021-00988-x

Borsari B, Yalch MM, Pedrelli P, Radomski S, Bachrach RL, Read JP (2018) Associations among trauma, depression, and alcohol use profiles and treatment motivation and engagement in college students. J Am Coll Heal 66(7):644–654. https://doi.org/10.1080/07448481.2018.1446438

Brave Heart MY (2003) The historical trauma response among natives and its relationship with substance abuse: a Lakota illustration. J Psychoactive Drugs 35(1):7–13. https://doi.org/10.1080/02791072.2003.10399988

Brave Heart MYH, Chase J, Elkins J, Altschul DB (2011) Historical trauma among indigenous peoples of the Americas: concepts, research, and clinical considerations. J Psychoactive Drugs 43(4):282–290. https://doi.org/10.1080/02791072.2011.628913

Cervantes RC, Gattamorta KA, Berger-Cardoso J (2019) Examining difference in immigration stress, acculturation stress and mental health outcomes in six Hispanic/Latino nativity and regional groups. J Immigr Minor Health 21(1):14–20. https://doi.org/10.1007/s10903-018-0714-9

Cypress BS (2021) Collective trauma: an evolutionary concept analysis. Nurs Forum (Hillsdale) 56(2):396–403. https://doi.org/10.1111/nuf.12550

Engel GL (1977) The need for a new medical model: A challenge for biomedicine. Science 196(4286):129–136. https://doi.org/10.1126/science.847460

Gone JP, Hartmann WE, Pomerville A, Wendt DC, Klem SH, Burrage RL (2019) The impact of historical trauma on health outcomes for indigenous populations in the USA and Canada: a systematic review. Am Psychol 74(1):20–35. https://doi.org/10.1037/amp0000338

Greenwood M, de Leeuw S, Lindsay NM (2018) Determinants of indigenous peoples' health, second edition: beyond the social. Canadian Scholars. https://play.google.com/store/books/details?id=jblaDwAAQBAJ, https://books.google.com/books/about/Determinants_of_Indigenous_Peoples_Healt.html?hl=&id=jblaDwAAQBAJ

Howard AE (2022) Transgenerational effects of trauma through epigenetic mechanisms. ProQuest Dissertations Publishing

Kira IA (2001) Taxonomy of trauma and trauma assessment. Traumatology 7(2):73–86. https://doi.org/10.1177/153476560100700202

Kira IA, Omidy AZ, Ashby JS (2014) Cumulative trauma, appraisal, and coping in Palestinian and American Indian adults: two cross-cultural studies. Traumatology 20(2):119–133. https://doi.org/10.1037/h0099397

Kira IA, Shuwiekh H, Al-Huwailah AH, Lewandowski L, Alawneh A-WN, Abou-Mediene S, Al Ibraheem B, Aljakoub J (2019) The central role of social identity in oppression, discrimination and social-structural violence: collective identity stressors and traumas, their dynamics and mental health impact. Peace Conflict 25(3):262–268. https://doi.org/10.1037/pac0000363

Lang AJ, Gartstein MA (2018) Intergenerational transmission of traumatization: theoretical framework and implications for prevention. J Trauma Dissociation 19(2):162–175. https://doi.org/10.1080/15299732.2017.1329773

Lehrner A, Yehuda R (2018) Cultural trauma and epigenetic inheritance. Dev Psychopathol 30(5):1763–1777. https://doi.org/10.1017/S0954579418001153

Liehr P, Smith MJ (2020) Claiming the narrative wave with story theory. Adv Nurs Sci 43(1):15–27. https://doi.org/10.1097/ANS.0000000000000303

Marmot M (2005) Social determinants of health inequalities. Lancet 365(9464):1099–1104. https://doi.org/10.1016/S0140-6736(05)71146-6

Marmot M (2018) Inclusion health: addressing the causes of the causes. Lancet 391(10117):186–188. https://doi.org/10.1016/S0140-6736(17)32848-9

Maxwell K (2014) Historicizing historical trauma theory: troubling the trans-generational transmission paradigm. Transcult Psychiatry 51(3):407–435. https://doi.org/10.1177/1363461514531317

Millender EI, Lowe J (2017) Cumulative trauma among Mayas living in Southeast Florida. J Immigr Minor Health 19(3):598–605. https://link.springer.com/article/10.1007/s10903-015-0337-3, https://link.springer.com/article/10.1007/2Fs10903-015-0337-3

Özlü-Erkilic Z, Wenzel T, Kothgassner OD, Akkaya-Kalayci T (2020) Transcultural differences in risk factors and in triggering Reasons of suicidal and self-harming behaviour in young people with and without a migration background. Int J Environ Res Public Health 17(18):6498. https://doi.org/10.3390/ijerph17186498

Power T, Wilson D, Best O, Brockie T, Bourque Bearskin L, Millender E, Lowe J (2020) COVID-19 and indigenous peoples: an imperative for action [report]. J Clin Nurs 29(15–16):2737. https://doi.org/10.1111/jocn.15320

Prevention, C. f. D. C. a (2022) What is epigenetics? Retrieved September, 29 from, https://www.cdc.gov/genomics/disease/epigenetics.htm

Sangalang CC, Becerra D, Mitchell FM, Lechuga-Peña S, Lopez K, Kim I (2019) Trauma, post-migration stress, and mental health: a comparative analysis of refugees and immigrants in the United States. J Immigr Minor Health 21(5):909–919. https://doi.org/10.1007/s10903-018-0826-2

Stanley K, Deirdre B (2019) Transgenerational trauma: the role of epigenetics. J Mind Behav 40(1):53–62

Stenz L, Schechter DS, Serpa SR, Paoloni-Giacobino A (2018) Intergenerational transmission of DNA methylation signatures associated with early life stress. Curr Genomics 19(8):665–675. https://doi.org/10.2174/1389202919666171229145656

Taylor J, Turner RJ (2002) Perceived discrimination, social stress, and depression in the transition to adulthood: racial contrasts. Soc Psychol Q 65:213–225

Taylor JY, Wright ML, Crusto CA, Sun YV (2016) The intergenerational impact of genetic and psychological factors on blood pressure (InterGEN) study: design and methods for complex DNA analysis. Biol Res Nurs 18(5):521–530. https://doi.org/10.1177/1099800416645399

Wilkinson R, Marmot M (1998) The solid facts: social determinants of health. Centre for Urban Health, World Health Organization. https://play.google.com/store/books/details?id=_ucqAAAACAAJ, https://books.google.com/books/about/The_Solid_Facts.html?hl=&id=_ucqAAAACAAJ

Yehuda R, Lehrner A, Bierer LM (2018) The public reception of putative epigenetic mechanisms in the transgenerational effects of trauma. Environ Epigenet 4(2):dvy018-dvy018. https://doi.org/10.1093/eep/dvy018

Zannas AS, Chrousos GP (2017) Epigenetic programming by stress and glucocorticoids along the human lifespan. Mol Psychiatry 22(5):640–646. https://doi.org/10.1038/mp.2017.35

Cumulative Trauma

8

Michelle Patch and Tamar Rodney

Objectives
- To describe cumulative trauma
- To explore the biopsychosocial effects of cumulative trauma
- To discuss therapeutic challenges and barriers to healing posed by cumulative trauma
- To explore nursing assessment and care approaches for individuals with cumulative trauma histories

Introduction

The causes of mental health disorders are complex and varied. Biological, psychological, and social factors are often interrelated in the role they play. Over a lifetime, individuals, families, and communities can experience multiple traumatic events. Determining the role of cumulative trauma exposure in the development of trauma-related health symptoms may also clarify the mechanisms underlying the observed variabilities in how individuals respond to traumatic events. The cumulative effects of these experiences and opportunities for healing will be the focus of this chapter.

The impact of cumulative trauma can have a wide range of psychological symptoms related to anxiety, depression, and post-traumatic stress disorder (PTSD). There is increasing evidence for a dose-response model in which stressors of greater severity, influenced by distance, repeated exposure, and duration, can lead to greater negative outcomes (Silver et al. 2021). Additionally, several factors specific to age

---

M. Patch (✉) · T. Rodney
Johns Hopkins University School of Nursing, Baltimore, MD, USA
e-mail: mpatch1@jhmi.edu; trodney1@jhu.edu

© The Author(s), under exclusive license to Springer Nature Switzerland AG 2025
T. Rodney (ed.), *Trauma Informed Care*,
https://doi.org/10.1007/978-3-031-87526-7_8

and cultural and societal norms may increase the risks and vulnerability to negative traumatic outcomes. These same factors also impact how we approach assessment, plan treatment goals, and support the health and well-being of individuals impacted by the cumulative burden of traumatic life events.

Acute Versus Chronic: Determines Official Diagnosis

The nature of trauma symptom presentation is variable. Acute stress and trauma encounters may develop and present symptoms in the first month after a traumatic event. There may, however, be a delay of months or years before symptoms start to appear. Some individuals can experience long periods when their symptoms are less noticeable, followed by periods in which they worsen. Presentation of symptoms may also be delayed for months to years (APA 2022). For trauma-related disorders, a clinical diagnosis requires an individual to "be exposed to: death, threatened death, actual or threatened serious injury, or actual or threatened sexual violence" (APA 2022). While this is often perceived as a singular event, individuals may be exposed to multiple events over a lifetime that can be experienced as traumatic.

Cumulative Trauma

Although the terms are frequently used interchangeably, cumulative trauma is understood to be distinctly different from generational trauma. Cumulative trauma (Fig. 8.1a) refers to additive exposure to traumatic events or experiences across an individual's lifetime (Cypress 2021). This contrasts with generational trauma (Fig. 8.1b), in which the effects of past traumatic experiences like war or oppression are unintentionally transmitted from parent to child.

How an individual interprets/perceives an event can influence the intensity of the trauma experienced. This can also influence the degree to which it interferes with their activities of daily living. Variability may also exist in the degree to which individuals experience distress or functional impairment *(DSM5-TR)*.

8 Cumulative Trauma

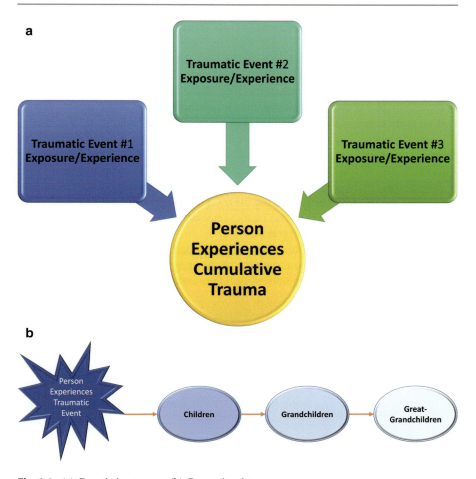

Fig. 8.1 (**a**) Cumulative trauma. (**b**) Generational trauma

Various Perspectives on Cumulative Trauma

According to the *biopsychosocial model* (Engel 1977), mental health is the result of many forces occurring at different time points, which have a cumulative effect on an individual. These influencing forces can be positive or negative (Silver et al. 2021). If the negatives exceed the positives, then a person could develop a mental illness. It is unlikely that one specific issue causes mental ill-health, but rather a combination of negative circumstances that have built up over time. There might be one thing that pushes a person too far, but it is unlikely to be this alone that causes a disorder.

Manifestations of traumatic experiences can also be examined within a *socio-ecological model* (Dahlberg and Krug 2002). This model explores how individual, relational, community, and societal factors intersect to influence the manifestations and outcomes of trauma (see Fig. 8.2).

The association between life stress and psychopathology has also been explored in various theoretical models. Examples of these explanatory/underpinning theories, which can give context to nurses' decision-making processes, are provided in Table 8.1.

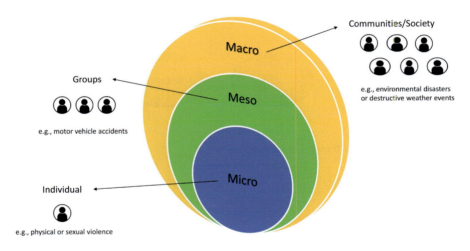

Fig. 8.2 Socio-ecological model

8 Cumulative Trauma

Table 8.1 Theoretical models

Model/hypothesis/theory	Definition	Examples
Diathesis-stress model AKA: Diathesis-stress hypothesis Diathesis-stress paradigm Diathesis-stress theory Stress-vulnerability model	"The theory that mental and physical disorders develop from a genetic or biological predisposition for that illness (diathesis) combined with stressful conditions that play a precipitating or facilitating role".	Depression: Monroe and Simons (1991) Schizophrenia: Bleuler (1963); Rosenthal (1960)
General adaptation syndrome	Pattern of bodily responses when exposed to demands from a stressor: (1) alarm; (2) adaptation; (3) exhaustion. Alarm, or "flight or fight", is the first reaction to a perceived threat. Physical changes include adrenal enlargement, thymicolymphatic involution, and gastrointestinal ulcers.	Selye (1936)
Adaptation model of nursing	"Adaptation occurs when people respond positively to environmental changes, and it is the process and outcome of individuals and groups who use conscious awareness, self-reflection, and choice to create human and environmental integration".	Roy and Andrews (1999)
Conservation of resource model	Those with increased access to resources are less vulnerable to stressors.	Hobfoll (2002)
Kindling hypothesis	Hypothesis "that life stressors may play an acute pathophysiological role in affective disorders and also serve as stimuli that lower the threshold of stress exposure necessary to trigger a recurrent episode. The kindling hypothesis thus states that initial episodes are likely triggered by major life events (stressors), but that successive episodes grow increasingly more autonomous".	Post (1992)
Theory of allostatic load	"Allostatic load refers to the cumulative burden of chronic stress and life events. It involves the interaction of different physiological systems at varying degrees of activity. When environmental challenges exceed the individual ability to cope, then allostatic overload ensues. Allostatic load is identified by the use of biomarkers and clinical criteria" (see Fig. 8.3).	McEwen and Stellar (1993); Guidi et al. (2021); Juster et al. (2010)
Stress generation hypothesis	"Depressive individuals are actively contributing to stressful environments, with the implication that such stressful conditions are likely to precipitate continuing or recurrent depression".	Hammen (2006)

(continued)

Table 8.1 (continued)

Model/hypothesis/theory	Definition	Examples
Association between stress and neurobiological systems related to reward	"A heuristic model...Postulating that anhedonia arises from dysfunctional interactions between stress and brain reward systems".	(Pizzagalli 2014)
Association between stress and neurobiological systems related to immune system inflammation: "Social signal transduction theory of depression"	"Hypothesis that experiences of social threat and adversity up-regulate components of the immune system involved in inflammation. The key mediators of this response, called *proinflammatory cytokines*, can in turn elicit profound changes in behavior, which include the initiation of depressive symptoms".	Slavich and Irwin (2014)
Association between stress and neurobiological systems related to corticosteroids	"Steroid hormone receptors also mediate rapid signaling pathways and, both direct and indirect genomic and non-genomic actions of steroids involve non-linear interactions with other intra- and extracelluar mediators. The resulting epigenetic effects result in ever-changing patterns of gene expression".	McEwen et al. (2016)

Additional theories that help to explain the body's response to events, often termed the "biology of trauma", include evidence related to the process of inflammation and a neutrophil-based reactionary process activated by the body. The innate immune response following a physical injury begins with neutrophils making a rapid and robust response against infection or harmful agents (Lehman and Segal 2020). While traditionally regarded as suicidal killers that cause collateral tissue damage, recent findings on neutrophil extracellular trap formation, heterogeneity, plasticity, and novel reparative functions have expanded our understanding of their diverse roles in health and disease. Advancing scientific insights into how neutrophils repair and regenerate tissue have helped to explain the unexpected aspects of neutrophils' involvement in regulating normal tissue homeostasis and its relationship to trauma (Wang 2018). Understanding the biology of trauma and cellular function, such as the role of neutrophils, can support a more holistic view of how the body's response contributes to inflammation and healing, offering new insights for trauma recovery.

The variability of an individual's experience of events can be influenced by the uniqueness of our individual backgrounds. Some people may be more disposed to develop a mental health issue than others, but we can all improve our mental health by seeing the biopsychosocial model as three positive forces for mental health. Focusing on the psychological aspects of the biopsychosocial model can empower people to take control of their thoughts and improve their mental health. Exploring an individual's background for their perceived strengths should inform diagnostic formulation as well as treatment planning.

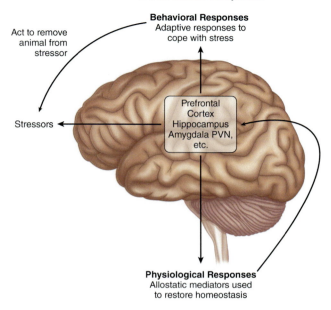
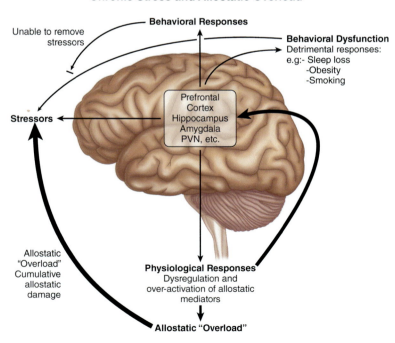

Fig. 8.3 Response to stressors. Central role of the brain in allostasis and the behavioural and physiological response to stressors. (With permission from McEwen (1998); Karatsoreos and McEwen (2010), Springer Nature)

Clinical Assessment, Diagnosis, Treatment Planning, and Implementation Considerations

Using the nursing process to guide care for patients with cumulative trauma, as illustrated in Fig. 8.4, provides significant value by ensuring a thorough, patient-centred approach. Initial assessment allows nurses to gather essential information about the patient's physical, emotional, and psychological state, considering the impact of cumulative trauma. This leads to an accurate *diagnosis*, identifying trauma-related conditions such as PTSD, anxiety, or depression. The *Treatment Planning* phase allows one to collaborate with patients to set specific, measurable goals focused on managing symptoms and promoting recovery. *Implementation Considerations* focus on utilizing evidence-based interventions, such as trauma-informed care and therapeutic approaches, while monitoring the patient's progress. The final step, *Evaluation*, allows one to assess whether the established goals are being met and whether adjustments are needed in the care plan, ensuring that the care remains responsive to the patient's evolving needs.

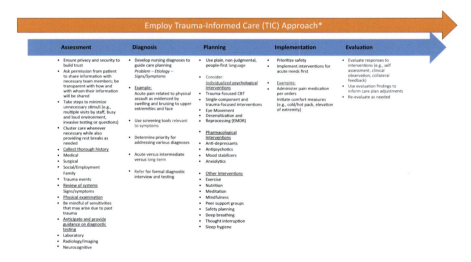

Fig. 8.4 Nursing process steps for patients with cumulative trauma

Table 8.2 The perspectives of psychiatry

Disease	Dimension	Behaviour	Life story
If you have gathered information about depressive symptoms, including neuro-vegetative symptoms, that goes in the column labelled disease	If you have gathered information about learning difficulties in school, that goes in the column labelled dimension	If you have gathered information about alcohol use, that goes in the column labelled behaviour	If you have gathered information about the death of a sibling in childhood, that goes in the column labelled life story. If you have gathered information about a family history of depression, that goes in column labelled disease and life story (e.g., if lived w/depressed mother)

Adapted from McHugh and Slavney (1998)

Perspectives of Psychiatry

The Perspectives of Psychiatry offers a structured way to explore an individual's experiences from four different vantage points (disease, dimensional, behaviour, and life story) (see Table 8.2). This provides an additional way for nurses to explore assessment and care approaches for individuals with cumulative trauma histories and offers a way of understanding the nature and origin of symptom presentations and a framework to build a care plan (McHugh and Slavney 1998).

Summary

Many individuals who experience trauma report being exposed to more than one traumatic event during their lifetime (APA 2022). The widespread prevalence of multiple lifetime traumas has driven interest in understanding the cumulative effects of exposure to trauma, given the potential for tailored treatment planning. There are multiple theories to guide clinicians' understanding of how cumulative trauma symptoms may present. An awareness of the varied impact of events and alignment of responses to an individual's experience should guide the approach to care planning.

Case

Sonya, a 22-year-old female, is in her second year of college and recently lost her neighbour who was a confidant and very close friend of the family. The impact has been profound on her, given her reports of an inability to concentrate, the near impossibility of studying for her final exams, and an overwhelming feeling of loss. Sonya shares that these feelings are like a series of unfortunate events over the last 6 years. On her 16th birthday, she witnessed the drowning death of her friend and the near death of her sister. Birthday celebrations have not been the same since, and she feels an overwhelming sense of guilt as she invited her friend along to celebrate that day. Prior to that, she lost her grandfather to a hit-and-run motor vehicle accident. She shares feeling vulnerable, broken, and not sure if she can cope. She recognizes that her behaviour towards her siblings has changed, and she feels alienated from her friends. She refuses to meet with her guidance counsellor or a therapist.

Discussion Questions

1. Can we heal from cumulative trauma?
2. How much trauma can an individual experience before they show signs of its effect?
3. How might the symptoms of cumulative trauma present differently among young adults?
4. Given the repeated experiences of death, how might we approach the assessment of trauma?
5. How might children who suffer trauma early in life show biological signs of ageing faster than children who have not?

Concepts
Allostasis
Cumulative trauma
Diathesis-stress model
Generational trauma
Perspectives of psychiatry
Stress related

References

APA (2022) DSM-5-TR(tm) classification. American Psychiatric Association Publishing
Bleuler M (1963) Conception of schizophrenia within the last fifty years and today [Abridged]. Proc R Soc Med 56(10):945–952
Cypress BS (2021) Collective trauma: an evolutionary concept analysis. Nurs Forum 56(2):396–403. https://doi.org/10.1111/nuf.12550

Dahlberg LL, Krug EG (2002) Violence: a global public health problem. In: Krug E, Dahlberg LL, Mercy JA, Zwi AB, Lozano R (eds) World report on violence and health. https://www.cdc.gov/violenceprevention/about/social-ecologicalmodel.html

Engel GL (1977) The need for a new medical model: a challenge for biomedicine. Science 196(4286):129–136. https://doi.org/10.1126/science.847460

Guidi J, Lucente M, Sonino N, Fava GA (2021) Allostatic load and its impact on health: a systematic review. Psychother Psychosom 90(1):11–27. https://doi.org/10.1159/000510696

Hammen C (2006) Stress generation in depression: reflections on origins, research, and future directions. J Clin Psychol 62(9):1065–1082. https://doi.org/10.1002/jclp.20293

Hobfoll SE (2002) Social and psychological resources and adaptation. Rev Gen Psychol 6(4):307–324. https://doi.org/10.1037/1089-2680.6.4.307

Juster RP, McEwen BS, Lupien SJ (2010) Allostatic load biomarkers of chronic stress and impact on health and cognition. Neurosci Biobehav Rev 35(1):2–16. https://doi.org/10.1016/j.neubiorev.2009.10.002

Karatsoreos IN, McEwen BS (2010) Stress and allostasis. In: Steptoe A (ed) Handbook of behavioral medicine. Springer, New York

Lehman HK, Segal BH (2020) The role of neutrophils in host defense and disease. J Allergy Clin Immunol 145(6):1535–1544. https://doi.org/10.1016/j.jaci.2020.02.038

McEwen BS (1998) Protective and damaging effects of stress mediators. N Engl J Med 338(3):171–179. https://doi.org/10.1056/nejm199801153380307

McEwen BS, Nasca C, Gray JD (2016) Stress effects on neuronal structure: hippocampus, amygdala, and prefrontal cortex. Neuropsychopharmacology 41(1):3–23. https://doi.org/10.1038/npp.2015.171

McEwen BS, Stellar E (1993) Stress and the individual. Mechanisms leading to disease. Arch Intern Med 153(18):2093–2101

McHugh PR, Slavney PR (1998) The perspectives of psychiatry. Wolters Kluwer Health, LWW

Monroe SM, Simons AD (1991) Diathesis-stress theories in the context of life stress research: implications for the depressive disorders. Psychol Bull 110(3):406–425. https://doi.org/10.1037/0033-2909.110.3.406

Pizzagalli DA (2014) Depression, stress, and anhedonia: toward a synthesis and integrated model. Annu Rev Clin Psychol 10:393–423. https://doi.org/10.1146/annurev-clinpsy-050212-185606

Post RM (1992) Transduction of psychosocial stress into the neurobiology of recurrent affective disorder. Am J Psychiatry 149(8):999–1010. https://doi.org/10.1176/ajp.149.8.999

Rosenthal D (1960) Confusion of identity and the frequency of schizophrenia in twins. Arch Gen Psychiatry 3(3):297–304. https://doi.org/10.1001/archpsyc.1960.01710030083011

Roy C, Andrews HA (1999) The Roy adaptation model. Prentice Hall

Selye H (1936) A syndrome produced by diverse nocuous agents. Nature 138:32

Silver RC, Holman EA, Garfin DR (2021) Coping with cascading collective traumas in the United States. Nat Hum Behav 5(1):4–6. https://doi.org/10.1038/s41562-020-00981-x

Slavich GM, Irwin MR (2014) From stress to inflammation and major depressive disorder: a social signal transduction theory of depression. Psychol Bull 140(3):774–815. https://doi.org/10.1037/a0035302

Wang J (2018) Neutrophils in tissue injury and repair. Cell Tissue Res 371(3):531–539. https://doi.org/10.1007/s00441-017-2785-7

Trauma Exposure and Symptom Presentations

Chitchanok Benjasirisan, Pearl Ed Cuevas, Veroina Deslandes, Rajesh Kumar, Tamar Rodney, Suratsawadee Kruahong, and Thitipong Tankampuan

Objectives
- Definition of the concept of trauma exposure
- Describe the different types of trauma exposure across the life span
- State the presentation of symptoms associated with trauma exposure across the life span
- Explain the association between trauma exposure and PTSD in the individual and family across the life span
- Design a plan of care for the individual, family, and community exposure to traumatic events or situations across the life span

---

C. Benjasirisan · T. Rodney · S. Kruahong
Johns Hopkins University School of Nursing, Baltimore, MD, USA
e-mail: cbenjas1@jhmi.edu; trodney1@jhu.edu; skruaho1@jhmi.edu

P. E. Cuevas
Centro Escolar University Manila, Manila, Philippines
e-mail: pegcuevas@ceu.edu.ph

V. Deslandes
University of the West Indies-Mona, Kingston, Jamaica
e-mail: veroina.deslandes@uwimona.edu.jm

R. Kumar
All India Institute of Medical Sciences, Rishikesh, Uttarakhand, India
e-mail: rajesh.nur@aiimsrishikesh.edu.in

T. Tankampuan (✉)
Mahidol University Faculty of Nursing, Bangkok, Thailand
e-mail: thitipong.tan@mahidol.ac.th

Introduction

The exposure of a person to traumatic events or situations, whether it be physiological or psychological or both, could have far-reaching consequences on the individual's quality of life. The objective of this chapter is to present an overview of trauma exposure and symptoms presentations to the individual, family, and community across the life span; also, to explore various coping strategies to deal with the effects of trauma exposure by the individual, family, and community across the life span. This chapter presented the experience of trauma among select groups around the world.

Trauma Exposure in Latin America and the Caribbean/Jamaica

In Latin America and the Caribbean (LAC), trauma exposure by its citizens is at an all-time high, with homicide being the leading cause of violent crime. Globally, Latin American and Caribbean countries, including Jamaica, have been referred to as one of the most violent regions, with one in four citizens perceiving crime and violence as the greatest threat to their security (Jaitman 2019). Violent crime against children, adolescents, and women is increasing and is a cause for public health concern.

In 2017, the homicide rate was 24 per 100,000 population (Jaitman 2019). Although LAC has less than 9% of the world's population, it accounts for 33.5% of the global homicide rate, three times more than the average world rate (UNODC, 2019 in Jaitman 2019). The study also revealed that violence against women and girls is pervasive in the region, with 29.8% of women experiencing physical and/or sexual intimate partner violence during their lifetime, which was more than the prevalence rate of 23.3% in North America. However, the prevalence rate for non-partner sexual violence was slightly less than in Africa, 10.7–11.9%, respectively.

The region's children are vulnerable to trauma exposure, whether physical, emotional, sexual, or neglect, and it requires all hands-on deck to save them. According to the World Health Organization (WHO), violence against children consists of all forms of violence against people under 18 years old perpetrated by family members, caregivers, peers, intimate partners, or strangers.

It is estimated globally that approximately one billion children between the ages of 2 and 17 have experienced some form of trauma yearly (WHO 2020a, b). Evidence shows that 58% of children in LAC have experienced some form of trauma (physical, psychological, sexual, neglect) during their lifetime (Guedes 2019).

Guedes (2019) reported that children between the ages of 1 and 14 years are at higher risk of experiencing violent discipline than children of older age.

Children exposed to violence risk long-term consequences on their health and well-being, eventually impacting families, communities, and nations. Evidence shows that violence against children can result in deaths, such as homicide, involving weapons such as firearms and knives and is among the top four causes of death in adolescents, with boys comprising over 80% of the victims and perpetrators (WHO 2020a, b).

Exposure to violence and other adversities at an early age for a child can interfere with the neurological and physiological developmental process and put them at risk of developing physical and mental health problems in adulthood (Kliethermes et al. 2014). The ACEs study by Felitti et al. (1998) on adverse childhood experiences and the effects on adult health status have demonstrated an increased risk for cancer, cardiovascular problems, emphysema, depression, substance use, and other behavioural problems.

There has been an increase in violence against children in Jamaica in recent times. According to Shetty (2020), four indicators may contribute to the dysfunction in adults, resulting in crime and violence, substance abuse, mental illnesses, teenage pregnancy, and unemployment, along with an increase in non-communicable diseases (diabetes, hypertension). He described these as poor parenting practices, poor psychosocial support, adverse childhood experiences, and unidentified untreated mental disorders in youth.

Research has shown that 8 out of 10 children aged 2–14 experience some form of violent discipline because of poor parenting practices due to corporal punishment, which is culturally condoned as a form of discipline in Jamaica (Shetty 2020). Also, poor communication between parents and children, and those children who are orphaned and made vulnerable to teenage pregnancies and early fatherhood.

United Nations Children's Fund (UNICEF) reported that 85% of Jamaican children under the age of 15 years experience physical and psychological violence in the home. In comparison, 6% under age 15 are subjected to severe disciplinary punishment by their caregivers. Similarly, children from a poor background are at higher risk of corporal discipline and neglect than children from a wealthy background (UNICEF 2019). Additionally, 1 out of 4 children is living in poverty, mostly in female-headed households and with disabilities. Children living in poverty are one and a half times more likely to access substandard water and sanitary facilities, three times more likely to be parents in their teenage years, three times more likely to have not been engaged by their fathers in their formative years, and most likely to be exposed to violent discipline.

The international community has recognized violence against women as a fundamental violation of human rights, embodying physical violence, emotional and verbal abuse, sexual and physical assault, humiliation, stalking, and sexual harassment by former or current intimate partners. Therefore, violence against women affects women of all ages, educational backgrounds, and socioeconomic statuses.

Intimate partner violence "refers to behavior by an intimate partner or ex-partner that causes physical, sexual or psychological abuse and controlling behavior" while *Sexual violence* is "any sexual act, attempt to obtain a sexual act, or other act directed against a person's sexuality using coercion", by any person regardless of the relationship to the victim, in any setting such as rape, attempted rape, unwanted sexual touching, and other non-contact forms, according to the World Health Organization (2021a, b).

Intimate partner violence (IPV) and sexual violence are among the most pervasive forms of violence against women and girls in Latin America and the Caribbean region. The World Health Organization estimated that 1 in 4 women aged between 15 and 49 years in Latin America and the Caribbean experience sexual or physical violence perpetrated by an intimate partner during their lifetime (WHO 2021a, b).

A study conducted by the United Nations among five Caribbean countries—Guyana, Suriname, Jamaica, Grenada, Trinidad, and Tobago—reveals that the prevalence of IPV against women was high. In addition, 49% of women see their role as to take care of the home, while 48% of women believe that it is natural for men to be the head of the family, and 60% of women experienced at least one controlling behaviour.

The detection of IPV symptoms is usually never recognized because victims fear their partners' reactions if they discover that they speak about the abuse. Similarly, they feel health professionals are judgemental towards them, so they would rather keep the abuse private among themselves, family members, and friends. Additionally, health professionals tend to regard violence against women as a legal issue or as a domestic matter; therefore, all categories of workers need to be sensitive towards responding to survivors of IPV (see Box 9.1 for symptoms of IPV).

Box 9.1: Symptoms of Intimate Partner Violence
Symptoms of Physical Violence

- Slapping, pushing, biting, hair pulling, throwing things, choking, kicking, burning, using, or threatening to use a weapon such as a gun or a knife

Symptoms of Sexual Violence

- Forced/coerced intercourse, intercourse out of fear, degrading or humiliating sex

Symptoms of Emotional Violence

- Prevented from seeing friends and/or family, insisting on knowing where she is at all times, verbal insults, making her feel scared or intimidated

General Signs and Symptoms Associated with IPV

- Depression, post-traumatic stress disorder, anxiety disorder, sleep difficulties, eating disorders, and suicide attempts
- Miscarriage, stillbirth, preterm delivery, and low birthweight babies
- Headache, pain syndrome (back pain, abdominal pain, chronic pelvic pain), gastrointestinal disorders, limited mobility, and poor overall health

Source: United Nations Survey 2016–2019

Factors associated with lifetime sexual and or physical intimate partner violence (IPV) span from a wide range of things, such as a partner who is controlling to poor communication, frequent quarrelling among the couple, women exposed to emotional abuse during childhood, women who are the main source of income and so these men feeling threatened, women who were beaten during childhood, partner uses recreational drugs at least once per week, partner has had extra-marital relationship, women educational level, women cannot speak freely to family or women who cannot count on family for support, women who have ever been pregnant, and a couple who do not talk about their day with each other (Haarr 2020).

The high incidence of crime and violence has severe repercussions on the social and economic development of countries in the region. Literature has quoted the cost of crime and violence to consume 3.5% of LAC's economic output (Jaitman 2019).

Plan of Care for a Child Sexually Abused

Plan of care	Child abuse
Assessment	The nurse ensures a therapeutic environment for the victim by being caring, accepting, and non-judgemental in obtaining detailed and sensitive information both subjectively and objectively about the case. The nurse or the health provider should ensure the observation of all protocols for reporting while maintaining privacy and confidentiality throughout the process
Diagnosis	Detailed data are critically analysed and synthesized of the clients' actual or potential needs. This is guided by the diagnostic and statistical manual, the fifth edition of psychiatric conditions
Planning	Setting goals or outcomes in terms of priority
Intervention	Once the goals are identified, strategies and alternatives are developed. Actions to be taken with the patient's input or involvement
Evaluation	This phase assesses how successful the outcomes were and what further actions may be needed for unmet needs

A Case of Sexual Assault

A child requires continuous guidance, protection, and security from their parents, relatives, friends, and the entire village to develop and adapt appropriately to childhood adversity. It is not easy to recognize a child who is sexually abused because the physical signs are not readily apparent, unlike in the case of physical abuse, where the symptoms are visible. Likewise, in some instances, the survivor is not able to explain what happened to them. On the other hand, the perpetrators often threaten to harm the victim's relatives or acquaintances if they should talk to anyone about the assault, which is a means of silencing the survivor. At the same time, he continues to carry out the assault unabated until he is caught. Sexual assault can happen to both males and females.

An 8-year-old girl had been sexually assaulted repeatedly, first by a male friend of the family and then by a relative. On the first occasion when she told her mother about her ordeal, nothing was done because her mother did not believe she was sexually abused. In some contexts, this is often the reaction of some parents or guardians when they first hear of the assault because either they are in denial or think the survivor is fabricating a story. Initially, she was infected with a sexually transmitted infection, which was treated. However, her second incident triggered a series of events that started in the home and then spilled into the school environment. She exhibited symptoms that were in keeping with empirical findings but are not pathognomonic to sexual assault only, such as aggression, frequent physical fights with the opposite sex, especially for minor things that do not warrant such behaviour, poor concentration, poor academic performance, socially withdrawn, and depression.

In caring for the patient, the nurse is faced with the challenging task of establishing a therapeutic alliance with the patient who may be experiencing mixed emotions and mistrust and, therefore, finds it difficult to cooperate during the assessment process. Thus, the healthcare provider must employ evidence-based knowledge and practices in the execution of trauma-informed care not only to the sexually assaulted survivor but also to the patient's mother, who is experiencing a strained relationship with her mother.

Critical Thinking Question

How should the nurse care for an adolescent who was sexually assaulted by a relative and who was accused of lying and wanted to create problems in the family but is now experiencing feelings of guilt, shame, low self-esteem, and hopelessness and does not trust anyone?

Trauma Exposure in Thailand

The concept of trauma exposure is defined as exposure to a traumatic incident or series of events that are frightening or upsetting. Individuals who have been exposed to trauma have been affected or threatened by an incident or series of events that are physically and psychologically distressing and that can have long-term negative effects on their functioning and physical, social, emotional, and/or spiritual well-being. Presentation of symptoms associated with types of trauma, including physical injury, psychotic episodes (i.e. hallucinations or delusion), depression, anxiety, mood disorders, and symptoms of post-traumatic stress disorder (PTSD).

In Thailand, the current study reported the relationship between trauma exposure and psychological alteration. The classification of traumatic events in Thailand was classified into three categories: (1) interpersonal traumatic event, i.e., beaten-up by someone else, civilian in a warzone, man-made disaster, sexually assaulted; (2) unintentional traumatic event, i.e., automobile accident, natural disaster, unintentionally life-threatening event, or death; and (3) not specified, i.e., not disclosed, witnessed death (Kilian et al. 2021). The participants in this study were Thai residents who were 18 years of age or older. According to the findings of the study, participants who had at least one experience with a traumatic incident were 2.3 times more likely to suffer from psychotic episodes than those who had no such experience. Furthermore, people who had encountered interpersonal traumatic events or accidental traumatic events were four times more likely to suffer from psychotic episodes than those who had not experienced trauma. Auditory hallucinations were the most prevalent psychotic episodes described by participants, followed by visual hallucinations, during the course of a lifetime.

This study examines the association between three distinct forms of trauma exposure and psychological alteration in Thai adults. In addition to that, there is a scenario in Thailand that poses a threat to Thai adults, particularly women. It is violence against women which is a major problem and global phenomenon, including in Thailand. There are several types of violence directed towards women. Intimate partner violence (IPV) and sexual violence (SV) are two of the most prevalent types.

Intimate partner violence is defined by the World Health Organization (2021a, b) as behaviour by an intimate partner or ex-partner that results in physical, sexual, or psychological harm, such as physical aggression, sexual coercion, psychological abuse, or controlling behaviours. The most recent prevalence study of IPV in Thailand interviewed 2462 married or cohabiting women aged 20–59 years about their experiences with psychologically, physically, sexually, and/or controlling behaviours by their male partners discovered that 15% of participants had experienced psychological, physical, and/or sexual violence in their lifetime, implying that one in every six Thai women has faced IPV (Chuemchit et al. 2018). Among the 15% of women who reported intimate partner violence over the previous 12 months, psychological violence was the most prevalent type of IPV (60–68%), followed by sexual violence (62–63%) and physical violence (52–65%) (Chuemchit et al. 2018). According to a study titled "Psychiatric disorders associated with intimate partner violence and sexual violence in Thai women", the lifetime experience of IPV exposure was associated with lifetime diagnoses of common mental illnesses, suicidal behaviours, and alcohol/illicit use disorders. There were also statistically significant relationships between lifetime SV experience and a current or former diagnosis of a mental illness or prior suicidal behaviour but not with a current or prior diagnosis of a substance use disorder (Panyayong et al. 2018). A study on violence against women and PTSD among female victims of former sex workers was conducted in Thailand's Nana Sukhumvit area and revealed that violence against women causes significant distress to mental health. Moreover, 91.7% of participants who experienced traumatic events acquired PTSD as a consequence of prolonged trauma-related issues (Petchtam 2019). Individuals who suffer from PTSD may have recurrent symptoms. Certain voices, images, scents, and ideas might stimulate one's memory of traumatic events. This process is referred to as triggers, which could bring vivid recollections of traumatic situations to the surface. While sharing their experiences, the majority of participants felt as though they were reliving traumatic events (Petchtam 2019). With PTSD, the individuals' brains neither immediately comprehend the traumatic events nor do they store the memory as being in the past. Consequently, individuals are always terrified and stressed, even when they are in a safe place (Petchtam 2019). IPV and SV are traumatic situations that can have substantial short- and long-term consequences for victims' physical, mental, sexual, and reproductive health. This also has an impact on their children's health and wellbeing. The adverse results of childhood IPV exposure include an increased risk of psychological, social, emotional, and behavioural problems in children and adolescents, including mood and anxiety disorders, post-traumatic stress disorder (PTSD), substance abuse, and school-related problems. As a result, doing a comprehensive examination of a patient's history of violence for patients of all ages would be recommended as effective in refining the diagnosis and treatment.

The other example of interpersonal traumatic events in Thailand is the long-lasting insurgency in deep southern Thailand, which encompasses three of the country's southernmost provinces and portions of a fourth. The insurgency began as a conflict between ethnic and religious separatists in the 1900s and escalated in complexity and violence in the early 2000s. Since then, violence and unprecedented attacks on innocent citizens have occurred, including a bomb outside a school, motorbike drive-by shootings, and detonations of improvised explosive devices. The violence peaked in 2007, with daily assaults resulting in an average of three deaths each day. In 2008, the Royal Thai Armed Forces sent a large number of personnel to the area, which aided in reducing the degree of violence, and 60,000 security forces remain in the region at the current day (Abuza 2015). There have been fewer attacks to date, and residents of the affected area continue to live relatively regularly. However, since the conflict is not yet resolved, random acts of violence may occur at any moment. People continue to reside there. However, a number of individuals relocate to different parts of the country to escape such a predicament. Multiple studies have shown that the people in affected areas suffer from PTSD and other mental health issues. Moreover, 37.2% of middle school children have experienced emotional and behavioural problems (Wichaidit 2018); 34.6% of soldiers deployed in Narathiwat Province tested positive for depression, while 19.7% reported significant alcohol use in the preceding month (Wichaidit 2018).

Additionally, there is a distinct instance of an unintentional traumatic event that occurred in Thailand. In 2004, an Indian Ocean tsunami, which are huge waves caused by earthquakes or volcanic eruptions under the water, hit the coasts of several countries in South and Southeast Asia, including Thailand. It killed approximately 280,000 people and destroyed buildings and infrastructure. Exposure to the tsunami disaster has a negative effect on both the physical and mental health of the people who lived there. A study that examined the impact of the 2004 tsunami on self-reported physical health in Thailand for the subsequent 2 years discovered that participants who suffered personal injury or lost business as a result of the tsunami reported poorer physical health than those who were unaffected, and greater negative impacts on health were shown in women and the elderly (Isaranuwatchai et al. 2013). Furthermore, a cohort study on the effect on mental health 1 and 2 years after tsunami exposure that investigated the association between six consequent variables (personal injury, loss of home, loss of business, death of a family member, injury to a family member, or loss of a family member's business) and mental health found that a year later, individuals who had been injured, lost a business, or lost a family member reported poorer mental health than those who had not been impacted. And, 2 years later, those who had lost a family member reported poorer mental health than those who had not (Isaranuwatchai et al. 2017). These studies emphasize the disaster's impact on the health of the population. PTSD and major depressive disorder (MDD) are the most prevalent mental health issues found after exposure to traumatic events, including natural disasters. There is no evidence for a difference in the presentation of symptoms across various ages following exposure to this incident in MDD. However, a focus group research conducted in Thailand's Phang-Nga area indicated that children exhibit distinct PTSD symptoms than adults (Downs and Othman 2015). The researchers classified invasive recall, hyperarousal, avoidant behaviours, and interpersonal problems as four PTSD symptom clusters. Hyperarousal and interpersonal problems were the most prevalent symptom clusters in children in the region, while adults had the fewest evident symptoms of interpersonal problems and invasive recall. Hyperarousal symptoms occurred more frequently than invasive recall, but at a rate less than half that of children, and adults exhibited a major increase in avoidant behaviours in comparison to other evident symptoms (Downs and Othman 2015).

Firefighters are subjected to physical and psychological stress on a daily basis in their work environment. This could be an example of individuals who experience occupational exposure to traumatic events. The presentation of symptoms associated with this type of trauma is found to be comparable to those associated with the other types. Khumtong and Taneepanichskul's (2019) research demonstrates a significant correlation between PTSD and sleep quality among Bangkok firefighters. PTSD was prevalent among firefighters at 6.4%, and more than 80% of individuals with PTSD had poor sleep quality. As a result, PTSD also appears to increase the probability of poor sleep quality among urban firemen in Thailand.

Plan of care	
1. Assessment	Trauma exposure, regardless of the type, can impact not just an individual's physical health but also their mental health. When evaluating someone who may have been exposed to or has been exposed to traumatic events, a thorough examination of the patient's history regarding any type of traumatic experience should be performed. Questions must be addressed to ascertain if symptoms are the result of a traumatic event or other mental diseases. The Diagnostic and Statistical Manual of Mental Disorders, Fifth Edition (DSM-5) can be used in conjunction with information gathered through thorough history taking to identify the patients' diagnosis and symptoms
2. Diagnosis	After assessing and identifying the patient, family, or community that are exposed to traumatic events, creating a list of the patient's problems through nursing diagnosis allows for a clear understanding of the issues that must be addressed
3. Planning	There is no fixed plan of care for each presentation of symptoms associated with various types of traumatic events. An individualized and tailored plan of care should be made to achieve the optimal outcome for each person, family, or community. Additionally, preventive intervention needs to be included in this process as well

(continued)

Plan of care		
4. Implementation	Most individuals who are exposed to traumatic events require a multidisciplinary approach involving nurses, physicians, psychologists, psychiatrists, social workers, and certified professional counsellors. Apart from assessing and delivering nursing care to patients, nurses can collaborate with other healthcare providers as case managers to manage, facilitate treatment, and advocate for patients as well
5. Evaluation	Once the plan is implemented, it is essential to conduct an evaluation to see whether the goals of care are being achieved. If not, the assessment process and other steps, respectively, are required

Case Study

You are a nurse vacationing in Phang-Nga, Thailand. On Sunday morning, you went on the speed boat to Phi Phi Island for snorkeling, and you were heading back to Khao Lak beach to go back to your hotel. While in the boat, you notice that the seawater has abruptly begun to recede. The boat driver is stunned and informs you and your group that "we cannot proceed to the shore at this time because something is not right". "It might be a tsunami similar to the one that occurred in 2004". Following the boat driver's words, one Thai woman on board begins to cry and screams, "This is not right". This is intolerable. Why is this occurring once more? Why, why, why? I simply wish to live a "happy life". Concurrently, there is a Royal Thai Navy ship that is far larger than the speed boat you are riding. The speedboat driver then requested assistance and evacuated everyone aboard the ship. The woman who was crying continued to cry. You learn throughout the talk on the way to Phi Phi Island that she travelled alone and wanted to visit since she missed her fiancée. In 2004, he proposed to her there, and the day after that, the tsunami attacked, and he went missing. Apart from the crying woman, the remaining three individuals, including the speed boat driver, appear nervous but are more composed.

What Would You Do as a Nurse?

Since there is a possibility that this is a tsunami, which is a sequence of massive waves that are potentially destructive and can endanger you and anybody else, the first step is to assess. You must first assess the circumstance and the environment in which you find yourself to determine whether they are safe for you and the other person. Being on board the large ship is safer than being on the shore, as the tsunami waves move towards the beach. Following that, it is necessary to assess and identify the patient. According to what you know about her, she has suffered a traumatic event in the past due to the loss of a loved one and is now confronted with a circumstance that reminds her of what happened. Thus, the following step is diagnosis. You may not have the resources or the time on the scene to perform the actual diagnostic test or questionnaire, but you would notice that she may be exhibiting PTSD symptoms.

And what you could do next is make a plan for the patient and implement it. This will be expedient if you are confronted with a real-world circumstance. Your goal should be to maintain the patient's safety and calmness and to be there for her. Do not leave her alone, and keep an eye out for any physical problems that may occur, such as hyperventilation, and if appropriate, ask about her past medical history and if she has been seeing a counsellor or psychiatrist. As a result, you would be able to ensure that she receives the necessary care. The evaluation process would also occur after the relaxation approach or any techniques used to soothe the patient. Additionally, you can refer her to a psychiatrist or counsellor following the incident.

Trauma Exposure in the Philippines

In the Philippines, the concept of trauma exposure was defined based on its physiological effect on the person. A dearth of literature discusses the psychological, mental, or psychosocial stress trauma brings to an individual. Some studies depict psychosocial trauma as a mental health concern leading to the hurt of oneself or others.

The Philippines is known to be one of the world's exporters of manpower, and some mental health concerns arise from this scenario. For the many Filipinos who work abroad, culture shock can lead to trauma. Problems with acculturation coupled with homesickness cause elevated mental health problem that also characterizes the Filipino overseas worker or migrants (Nguyen and Bornheimer 2014). It is estimated that around 12% of US-based Filipinos suffer from psychological distress (Nicdao et al. 2015). This is relatively higher than the US prevalence rate for depression and anxiety (WHO 2017). A report released by the World Health Organization has estimated that the overall prevalence of depression in the Philippines was 3.3%, suggesting that about 3.3 million Filipinos experience depressive symptoms based on the 2015 population estimate of the Philippine Statistics Authority.

Mental illness was the third most common disability in the Philippines. Around six million Filipinos were estimated to live with depression or anxiety, making the Philippines the country with the highest rate of mental health problems in the Western Pacific region. Depression can lead to suicide, and the rates were pegged at about 2.2 per 100,000 population (2019), while the numbers can possibly be higher due to underreporting or misclassification of suicide cases as "undetermined deaths" (Redaniel et al. 2011). This was more so during the pandemic because end-of-life attempts were reported to be attributed to a positive COVID diagnosis, helplessness, hopelessness, anxiety, hunger, and depression.

For the many Filipino overseas workers, the long periods of family separation and being exposed to a different cultural background can make each Filipino family member prone to trauma, acculturative stress, depression, anxiety, and even substance use, especially those who are exposed to abuse, violence, and discrimination while overseas (Green and Ayalon 2016).

Post-traumatic stress disorder (PTSD) is one of the most common mental health disorders in the Philippines (Theisen-Womersley 2021). Research indicates that PTSD cases typically rise following natural disasters, such as the eruption of Mt. Pinatubo in 1991(Howard et al. 1999) and the devastation caused by Typhoon Yolanda in 2013 (Horiguchi and Nakazawa 2021). PTSD cases have also been reported in regions affected by armed conflict, insurgency, and within military personnel, where the prevalence tends to rise (Ahmed et al. 2024).

However, a barrier to Filipinos exposed to trauma was the propensity to not seek psychological help (Ho et al. 2018; Bernardo and Estrellado 2017). Compared to other minority Asian groups, Filipino rates were low and even much lower than the general US population (Kessler et al. 2007; Abe-Kim et al. 2007). Factors that may be associated with this were attributed to the loss of face, stigma tolerance, and acculturation factors (Tuliao 2014 & Gong et al. 2003).

Both local and overseas Filipinos indicated that professional help was sought only as a last resort because they were more inclined to get help from the community, families, friends, or lay network (Ho et al. 2018; Vahabi and Wong 2017).

Although the Philippines reported the five most common recorded trauma exposures as physiological in nature as related to open wound(s), superficial injury of any part of the body, fracture of the hand, minor traumatic brain injury, and fracture of the patella, tibia or fibula, or ankle (Rivera et al. 2018). The Philippines were also victim to events and situations that can lead to the development of psychological and/or psychosocial trauma. These may include natural disasters such as fires, floods, storm surges, earthquakes, volcanic eruptions, and massive ash falls. On an interpersonal level, violence like rape, child abuse, or the suicide of a loved one or friend was also considered as a traumatic incident.

In this country, suicide and gaming disorders were also identified as among the major social issues leading to psychological trauma. The common circumstances correlated with mental health concerns in the youth were too much academic pressure with great difficulty balancing time. This was coupled with excessive use of digital devices, engaging in network gaming and social media, as these can lead to depression, breakdown of personal connectedness, and cyberbullying. The Philippines, being one of the most active users of social media sites (Pond et al. 2020), pose a risk of adolescent addiction and depression.

In times of disasters, children and adolescents also experience a wide range of mental and behavioural trauma shown in disturbances such as sleeplessness, fear, anxiety, depression, and even post-traumatic stress disorder (Kar 2009). Children with experiences in evacuation centres and living in temporary housing shelters had externalization symptoms and concerns. Also affecting the children were economic disparities, parents' mental state, and less social support. The care for disabled children after disasters was also a challenge, as children with Autism have difficulty adjusting to the crowded evacuation centres (Estrada et al. 2020). More so, in the Philippines, evacuation centres were swarming with people after a disaster. This collectively affects the mental health of the children, adolescents, and their families.

Child abuse in the country takes the form of online child sexual exploitation and substance abuse. The Philippines was one of the top sources of child pornography material (UNICEF 2020a), and this has been reported as an emerging social issue in the country. Since an increasing trend in sexual abuse has been observed, physical abuse was likely to be underreported. Even so, corporal punishment was commonly an accepted method of disciplining Filipino children. Surprisingly, psychological abuse was least recognized and reported in the country, even though a national baseline study found that 3 of 5 children experience it (UNICEF 2020b). Thus, medical and psychosocial care for abused women and children in the Philippines must be made timely and relevant.

A recommendation for multidisciplinary teams to manage individual cases of trauma (Estrada et al. 2020) was advocated. The team may be composed of psychiatrists, social workers, nurses, and occupational therapists.

In child abuse, nurses and social workers can serve as case managers. These professionals can be trained in many different forms of psychotherapy, such as Trauma-focused Cognitive Behavioural Therapy (TF-CBT), defined as evidence-based psychotherapy or counselling that aims at addressing the needs of children and adolescents with post-traumatic stress disorders and other difficulties related to traumatic life events.

Plan of care	
1. Assessment	Upon assessment, the nurse must be mindful of culturally sensitive nursing care. Remember that when performing the IPPA: Filipinos may not be comfortable to disclose information to a stranger, so having someone in the room with whom the patient is comfortable can be quite helpful. A family member or friend should usually be present Filipinos do not respond easily to straightforward questioning, so the nurse must allot time to develop trust Asking permission to touch the patient or to talk about sensitive issues may be necessary For patients reluctant to seek help, remind them of their rights and responsibilities Let the Diagnostic and Statistical Manual of Mental Disorders, Fifth Edition (DSM-5) guide the nurse in the trauma or mental illness assessment
2. Diagnosis	Nursing diagnosis takes into account the cultural response of the patient related to the trauma encountered. Diagnoses were based on immediate needs such as safety, physiological health, and mental security
3. Planning	Plan with the patient to take into consideration her own time frame It would also be beneficial to include family members when planning for care since Filipinos see self in the context of their family
4. Implementation	When implementing culturally sensitive nursing care, it is important to understand how the patient sees herself and her relationship to the environment. Patient actions are not usually individualistic but collective as her decisions affect that of family members
5. Evaluation	It is important to evaluate with the patient the plan and course of action to be undertaken. Trauma may take more time to address; therefore, careful re-evaluation of the care plan is deemed necessary. Nurses can write continuous nursing care plans until the patient has reached the goal

Case Study

Alicia lived in a mansion at the foot of Lake Taal and Volcano in Batangas, Philippines. Her family was said to be well off as they lived in a big house and had a herd of farm animals. They also have a vegetable plantation in their huge backyard.

When the Taal Volcano erupted, their area suffered the hardest hit. Tons of Ash fall buried their house and most of the houses in the community. As Alicia started to run away with her two children towards the road to safety, she could only see the rooftop of her home. At the sight of this, she felt doomed. Then panic struck; she realized that she was not able to bring anything but all she knew was that she wanted to save the life of her two children and bring them to safety.

Her husband, Rommel, ran back towards their home to try and save their livestock. Although Alicia called to him, he persisted, and midway to the fields, she saw him fall to the ground, choking in ash and unable to breathe. His last words were, "Go save our children, Leave me here". As Alicia shouted and cried in anguish, she saw her husband, their farm, plantation, and home turn into a white pile of mud. She realized then that her children must be taken to safety, so she went and spared no time to grieve her loss. As she ran with nothing but her children, she felt the sense of doom envelope her and knew that almost everything she worked hard for had been taken away from her.

Alicia walked for miles and miles until about 6 h passed when she reached the evacuation centre, too tired from carrying her two children who had been passed out from the journey. The centre was an old school building cramped with so many families, crying or wailing in pain. She overheard someone saying, "The roads are covered with ash falls! It will take days before rescue workers can come in to find us! We do not have enough food or water". At this time, Alicia clutched her children tightly and braved to ask people in the evacuation centre if they could spare them a piece of bread and some water for her children.

But Alicia and her children starved for days in a building corner overflowing with people until help finally came. In the past week, she has seen many people die of hunger and sickness in the evacuation area. She wondered if she would be able to live long enough to look after her children.

When a psychological first aider came to talk to her, she was already staring blankly into space. How can she even begin to tell her story?

As a Nurse, How Can You Help This Patient?

Alicia, now a single parent, must brave the world on her own. She must learn to be resilient to be able to stand up again and raise her two children. According to the society-to-cells framework, the resilience potential of each human being needs to be the essential focus of our nursing care (Szanton and Gill 2010).

Initially, the major concern of Alicia was the safety of her children. However, as a nurse, you collectively see the family, and all of them must be taken into safety. Alicia honoured her husband's last request to take care of her children, and she needs to be strong to do this. She must see herself within the context that her children need her to be well so that together they can survive hardships that may follow. Recognizing this could affect her will and motivation to move on and get better, as well as her ability to be resilient.

As nurses, we see the family as a collective whole, and at the present time, the priority is to place them in an environment that promotes healing. A therapeutic milieu with clean air to breathe and adequate lighting for examination to check what they sustained during the trauma.

Initially, offering them physiologic nourishment is essential. Food and hydration are important for energy and sustenance, along with an adequate amount of rest.

When the body is ready, we can institute psychological first aid to determine the kind of healing needed by the family. As holistic beings, the needs of their mind, body, and spirit must be addressed to be able to harness their coping abilities.

Trauma Exposure in India

A variety of reactions are often observed and/or reported by trauma victims. However, these reactions might be acute or chronic in nature and depend on the vulnerability of trauma victims. Furthermore, the response pattern depends on individualized resilience status and the use of appropriate coping mechanisms, including social support and aftermath situation. However, a majority of trauma victims recover without any sign of distress and function festively in different life domains (SAMHSA 2014).

India is expecting a huge burden of road traffic-related post-traumatic stress disorder in future. There is a crisis in large-scale data on different psychiatric issues in post-trauma patients. However, a survey from the national capital reported symptoms of post-traumatic stress disorders in more than two-thirds of earthquake victims (Chadda et al. 2007). Similarly, 14% of women who reported intimate partner violence reported post-traumatic stress disorder (PTSD) and depressive symptoms (Chandra et al. 2009). Likewise, patients with higher burn reported more psychological symptoms, including acute stress disorder, depression, suicidal ideation, and post-traumatic stress disorder (Dalal et al. 2010). Furthermore, the prevalence of psychological disorders is often high in bomb blast trauma victims, who report acute stress reaction, depression, dissociative amnesia, sleep disturbances, nightmares, guilt, self-blame, and suicidal ideation (Gautam et al. 1998). However, the occurrence of psychological disorders is not time-specific and needs more robust data on this aspect.

Role of Nurse in Trauma Prevention and Treatment in India

The role of nurses in trauma is wide and begins with the prevention to rehabilitation of trauma victims. Trained trauma nurses play an essential role in the sensitization of the community on various aspects of trauma and help them to understand the analogy of trauma and its consequences. Trauma does not affect an individual but brings physical and psychological impacts on family members and relatives. A nurse should help in spreading awareness on different and common causes of trauma and their prevention. Nurses are in a key position to make the public aware of prevention acts, quick injury identifications, and laws and acts on prevention and assist the trauma victims to prevent injury and deaths (National Academies of Sciences, Engineering, and Medicine et al. 2021).

Promoting Injury Prevention

Injury is the leading cause of death and disability in children and adolescents. Trauma nurses are at the forefront to receive and intervene for trauma victims. Within the last few years, the role of nurses has shifted to the prevention of injury and educating more on preventive acts. Education of parents and children at trauma settings and the community level has an important, far-reaching effect on the prevention of injury. Wring in newspapers, blogs, use of social media, radio, and other sources could be alternative sources to educate the community at a personal level (Chen and Wang 2021). Use of clear and simple language without medical jargon will make the education effective at the grassroots level.

Advocacy in Trauma

Advocacy is another important role trauma nurses can play. In advocacy, a nurse focuses on keen assessment of the patient's need and ensures safe patient care throughout the trauma interventions. Advocacy can begin at the community level to make the people aware of their rights and raise their voice for any nontangible acts against them (The Role of the Trauma Nurse in Injury Prevention & Outreach). One example includes trauma nurses partnering with community leaders to raise awareness about the risks of consuming spurious liquor (hooch), aiming to reduce episodic overdoses through education, outreach, and proactive prevention efforts.

Trauma-Informed Care (TIC)

Trauma nurses deliver patient-centred care to improve quality and satisfaction. Trauma-informed care helps nurses to provide trusting, emotionally supportive, and collaborative care. TIC not only helps to deliver efficient care but also helps to attain the distinct experience of trauma survivors. Furthermore, trauma-informed care helps revise policy and framework to ensure safe settings and services to patients and staff. The use of clear communication while maintaining interpersonal reactions to empower patients and other staff is one of the benefits of trauma-informed care

(Substance Abuse and Mental Health Services Administration [SAMHSA] 2014). TIC helps to focus on what has happened to this person over time rather than 'what is wrong with this person' (Williamson and Kautz, 2018).

Counselling in Trauma Rehabilitation

Trauma rehabilitation is a complex process and may require repeated training and education to restore the activity of daily living and social integration. Trauma recovery requires an integrated approach, from individual counselling to changes in the physical and social environment (Williamson and Kautz 2018). However, a lack of trained trauma nurses in resource-driven countries, including India, is thought to be a contributing factor towards the lack of participation by trauma nurses.

Discussion Questions

1. What do you think about the different cultural responses to the trauma experience?
2. In the context of some cultures, in which most women believe they have less power than men, what would you do as a nurse to encourage a woman who is experiencing intimate partner violence (IPV) but is afraid to report it to the police because she believes it will only cause her more trouble?

References

Abe-Kim J, Takeuchi DT, Hong S, Zane N, Sue S, Spencer MS et al (2007) Use of mental health–related services among immigrant and US-born Asian Americans: results from the National Latino and Asian American study. Am J Public Health 97(1):91–98

Abuza Z (2015) The smoldering Thai insurgency CTC Sentinel 8(6):8–11

Ahmed SH, Zakai A, Zahid M, Jawad MY, Fu R, Chaiton M (2024) Prevalence of post-traumatic stress disorder and depressive symptoms among civilians residing in armed conflict-affected regions: A systematic review and meta-analysis. Gen Psychiatry. 37(3):e101438. https://doi.org/10.1136/gpsych-2023-101438

Bernardo AB, Estrellado AF (2017) Locus-of-hope and help seeking intentions of Filipino women victims of intimate partner violence. Curr Psychol 36(1):66–75

Chadda RK, Malhotra A, Kaw N, Singh J, Sethi H (2007) Mental health problems following the 2005 earthquake in Kashmir: Findings of community-run clinics. Prehosp Disaster Med. 22(6):541–546. https://doi.org/10.1017/s1049023x00005409

Chandra PS, Satyanarayana VA, Carey MP (2009) Women reporting intimate partner violence in India: Associations with PTSD and depressive symptoms. Arch Womens Ment Health. 12(4):203–209. https://doi.org/10.1007/s00737-009-0065-6

Chen J, Wang Y (2021) Social media use for health purposes: Systematic review. J Med Internet Res. 23(5):e17917. https://doi.org/10.2196/17917

Chuemchit M, Chernkwanma S, Rugkua R, Daengthern L, Abdullakasim P, Wieringa SE (2018) Prevalence of intimate partner violence in Thailand. J Fam Violence 33(5):315–323. https://doi.org/10.1007/s10896-018-9960-9

Dalal PK, Saha R, Agarwal M (2010) Psychiatric aspects of burn. Indian J Plast Surg. 43(Suppl):S136–S142. https://doi.org/10.4103/0970-0358.70731

Downs LL, Othman PSAP (2015) The incidence of posttraumatic stress symptoms among adults and children in the Phang Nga Region of Thailand

Estrada CA, Usami M, Satake N, Gregorio E Jr, Leynes C, Balderrama N, Fernandez de Leon J, Concepcion RA, Timbalopez C, Tsuji N, Harada I, Masuya J, Kihara H, Kawahara K, Yoshimura Y, Hakoshima Y, Kobayashi J (2020) Current situation and challenges for mental health focused on treatment and care in Japan and The Philippines- highlights of the training program by the National Center for Global Health and medicine. BMC Proc. (Open Access Meeting Report). 11–13 September 2019. 5-7 November 2019

Felitti VJ, Anda RF, Nordenberg D et al (1998) Relationship of childhood abuse and household dysfunction to many of the leading causes of death in adults. The adverse childhood experiences (ACEs) study. Am J Prev Med 14(4):245–258

Gong F, Gage SL, Tacata LA Jr (2003) Helpseeking behavior among Filipino Americans: a cultural analysis of face and language. J Community Psychol 31(5):469–488

Gautam S, Gupta ID, Batra L, Sharma H, Khandelwal R, Pant A (1998) Psychiatric morbidity among victims of bomb blast. Indian J Psychiatry. 40(1):41–45.

Green O, Ayalon L (2016) Whom do migrant home care workers contact in the case of work-related abuse? An exploratory study of help-seeking behaviors. J Interpers Violence 31(19):3236–3256

Guedes A (2019) Violence against children in Latin America and the Caribbean: Data and action. Pan American Health Organization. Available from: https://www.paho.org/sites/default/files/2023-11/violence-against-children-lac-keynote-guedes-2019.pdf

Haarr R (2020) Research brief-intimate partner violence in five CARICOM countries: findings from national prevalence surveys on violence against women. 20201009 CARICOM Research Brief 5.pdf (unwomen.org)

Ho GW, Bressington D, Leung SF, Lam K, Leung A, Molassiotis A et al (2018) Depression literacy and health-seeking attitudes in the Western Pacific region: a mixed-methods study. Soc Psychiatry Psychiatr Epidemiol 53(10):1039–1049

Horiguchi H, Nakazawa M (2021) Long-lasting effects of the 2013 Yolanda typhoon on overall health of mothers and children. Disaster Med Public Health Prep. 15(3):344–351. https://doi.org/10.1017/dmp.2020.40

Howard WT, Loberiza FR, Pfohl BM, Thorne PS, Magpantay RL, Woolson RF (1999) Initial results, reliability, and validity of a mental health survey of Mount Pinatubo disaster victims. J Nerv Ment Dis187(11):661–672. https://doi.org/10.1097/00005053-199911000-00003

Isaranuwatchai W, Coyte PC, McKenzie K, Noh S (2013) Impact of the 2004 tsunami on self-reported physical health in Thailand for the subsequent 2 years. Am J Public Health 103(11):2063–2070. https://doi.org/10.2105/ajph.2013.301248

Isaranuwatchai W, Coyte PC, McKenzie K, Noh S (2017) The 2004 tsunami and mental health in Thailand: a longitudinal analysis of one-and two-year post-disaster data. Disasters 41(1):150–170

Jaitman L (2019) Frontiers in the economics of crime: lessons for Latin America and the Caribbean. Lat Am Econ Rev 28:19. https://doi.org/10.1186/s40503-019-0081-5

Kar N (2009) Psychological impact of disasters on children: review of assessment and interventions. World J Pediatr 5(1):5–11

Kessler RC, Angermeyer M, Anthony JC et al (2007) Lifetime prevalence and ageof-onset distributions of mental disorders in the World Health Organization's world mental health survey initiative. World Psychiatry 6:168–176

Khumtong C, Taneepanichskul N (2019) Posttraumatic stress disorder and sleep quality among urban firefighters in Thailand. Nat Sci Sleep 11:123–130. https://doi.org/10.2147/nss.S207764

Kilian C, Supanya S, Probst C, Morgan C, Bärnighausen T, Kittirattanapaiboon P, Kwansanit P, Reininghaus U (2021) Traumatic events and psychotic experiences: a nationally representative study in Thailand. Epidemiol Psychiatr Sci 30:e47. https://doi.org/10.1017/S2045796021000172

Kliethermes M, Schact M, Drewry K (2014) Complex trauma. Child Adolesc Psychiatric Clin N AM 23:339–361

National Academies of Sciences, Engineering, and Medicine; National Academy of Medicine; Committee on the Future of Nursing 2020–2030; Flaubert JL, Le Menestrel S, Williams DR, et al. The Future of Nursing 2020-2030: Charting a Path to Achieve Health Equity. Washington (DC): National Academies Press (US); 2021. Nurses in disaster preparedness and public health emergency response. Available from: https://www.ncbi.nlm.nih.gov/books/NBK573904/

Nguyen D, Bornheimer LA (2014) Mental health service use types among Asian Americans with a psychiatric disorder: considerations of culture and need. J Behav Health Serv Res 41(4):520–528

Nicdao EG, Duldulao AA, Takeuchi DT (2015) Psychological distress, nativity, and help-seeking among Filipino Americans. In: Education, social factors, and health beliefs in health and health care services. Emerald Group Publishing Limited, pp 107–120

Panyayong B, Tantirangsee N, Bogoian RRD, Thai National Mental Health Survey, T (2018) Psychiatric disorders associated with intimate partner violence and sexual violence in Thai women: Aresult from the Thai National Mental Health Survey. General psychiatry 31(2):e000008. https://doi.org/10.1136/gpsych-2018-000008

Petchtam K (2019) Violence against women: PTSD in female victims of the former sex Workers in Nana Sukhumvit Area, Thailand. International Journal of Crime, Law and Social Issues 6(2). https://doi.org/10.2139/ssrn.3546348

Pond R, Leeding G, Ryan Dubras W-DD (2020) Digital 2020: 3.8 billion people use social media [Internet]. We Are Social [cited 2020 Mar 10]. Available from: https://wearesocial.com/blog/2020/01/digital-2020-3-8-billion-peopleuse-social-media

Redaniel MT, Lebanan-Dalida MA, Gunnell D (2011) Suicide in The Philippines: time trend analysis (1974–2005) and literature review. BMC Public Health 11(1):536

Rivera A, Lam H, Macalino J (2018) Epidemiology of injuries in The Philippines: an analysis of secondary data. Acta Med Philipp 52(2):180–186

SAMHSA (2014) SAMHSA concept of trauma and guidance for a trauma-informed approach. SAMHSA's Concept of Trauma and Guidance for a Trauma-Informed Approach (hhs.gov)

Shetty G (2020) Mental health conference 2020-day 4. https://www.youtube.com/watch?v=27JeeMApfj8

Substance Abuse and Mental Health Services Administration (SAMHSA) (2014) Effects of trauma. U.S. Department of Health and Human Services. Available from: https://www.samhsa.gov

Szanton S, Gill J (2010) Facilitating resilience using a society-to-cells framework: a theory of nursing essentials applied to research and practice. ANS Advance Nursing Science 33(4):329–343. https://doi.org/10.1097/ANS.0b013e3181fb2ea2

Theisen-Womersley G (2021) Prevalence of PTSD among displaced populations—Three case studies. In: Trauma and resilience among displaced populations. Springer; p. 41–57. https://doi.org/10.1007/978-3-030-67712-1_3

Tuliao AP (2014) Mental health help seeking among Filipinos: a review of the literature. Asia Pac J Couns Psychother 5(2):124–136

UNICEF (2020a) Philippines. A Systematic Literature Review of the Drivers of Violence Affecting Children in the Philippines [Internet]. UNICEF Philippines; 2016 [cited 23 March 2020]. Available from: https://www.unicef.org/philippines/media/506/file/National%20Baseline%20Study%20on%20Violence%20Against%20Children%20in%20the%20Philippines:%20Systematic%20literature%20review%20of%20drivers%20of%20violence%20affecting%20children%20(executive%20summary).pdf

UNICEF (2020b) Council for the Welfare of Children, UNICEF Philippines. National Baseline Study on Violence Against Children: Philippines Executive Summary [Internet]. 2016 [cited 23 March 2020]. Available from: https://www.unicef.org/philippines/media/491/file/National%20Baseline%20Study%20on%2Violence%20Against%20Children%20in%20the%20Philippines:%20Results%20(executive%20summary).pdf

United Nations Children's Fund (UNICEF) (2019) A statistical profile of violence against children in Latin America and the Caribbean. UNICEF. Available from: https://www.unicef.org/jamaica/media/2801/file/Violence%20Booklet_compressed.pdf.pdf

Vahabi M, Wong JP (2017) Caught between a rock and a hard place: mental health of migrant live-in caregivers in Canada. BMC Public Health 17(1):498

WHO (2017) Mental health atlas 2017, vol 2. World Health Organization

WHO (2020a) Child and adolescent mental health [Internet]. World Health Organization [cited 2020 Mar 06]. Available from: https://www.who.int/mental_health/maternal-child/child_adolescent/en/

WHO (2020b) Mental health action plan 2013–2020 [Internet]. World Health Organizations; 2013 [cited 2020 Mar 10]. Available from https://apps.who.int/iris/bitstream/handle/10665/89966/9789241506021_eng.pdf;jsessionid=3E09FA457C31F4CAF837E14AD6FD2B18?sequence=1

Wichaidit W (2018) Trauma from armed conflict and the effect on mental health in Thailand's deep south: a systematic review. Journal of Clinical & Diagnostic Research 12(7):VE01–VE06. https://doi.org/10.7860/jcdr/2018/35017.11722

Williamson LF, Kautz DD (2018) Trauma-informed care is the best clinical practice in rehabilitation nursing. Rehabil Nurs. 43(2):73–80. https://doi.org/10.1097/RNJ.0000000000000091

World Health Organization (2021a) Violence against women. https://www.violenceag-ainst-women (who.int)

World Health Organization (2021b) Violence against women. Retrieved March 11, 2022 from https://www.who.int/news-room/fact-sheets/detail/violence-against-women

Trauma Assessment

10

Tamar Rodney and Emma Mangano

Objectives
- Describe the nursing assessment approach for trauma exposure across the lifespan
- Identify validated screening and diagnostic tools for assessing trauma across the lifespan
- Discuss nursing interventions for trauma and application across the lifespan
- Identify the role of the nurse in initiating trauma-informed assessments and the referral process

Introduction

Trauma assessment is a critical first step for individuals, and there are multiple considerations that should inform the process. A trauma-informed approach guides one to consider the "Four Rs". Firstly, *realize* that an event has occurred that may have been traumatic for an individual and their community and the potential widespread impact; *recognize* the variability of symptom presentations of trauma; *respond,* by appropriately utilizing knowledge into policies practices and procedures and actively resisting any traumatization of that individual; and *resisting re-traumatization* for both the evaluee and evaluator by maintaining a therapeutic environment (SAMHSA 2014). This extends to the selection of the appropriate tool to guide the assessment process based on age, setting, and sensitivity to time and traumatic events.

T. Rodney · E. Mangano (✉)
Johns Hopkins University School of Nursing, Baltimore, MD, USA
e-mail: trodney1@jhu.edu; ebarth3@jhmi.edu

© The Author(s), under exclusive license to Springer Nature Switzerland AG 2025
T. Rodney (ed.), *Trauma Informed Care*,
https://doi.org/10.1007/978-3-031-87526-7_10

Nursing Assessment

As nurses, the evaluation of patients with a known, suspected, or unknown history of trauma should be approached using the nursing process. The American Nurses Association (ANA) describes this as a way to unite all nurses, despite the area they work in, in a single process; it provides nurses with the steps to deliver holistic, patient-focused care (ANA 2022). The nursing process includes five essential steps, although some may find it described in four or six steps. This includes an assessment, diagnosis, planning, implementation, and evaluation (Table 10.1). Since this is the core to nursing practice, these concepts will be discussed briefly as a review.

When assessing for trauma, nurses will need to review all available evidence to help guide their care going forward. This will include utilizing screening and diagnostic tools, head-to-toe evaluations for bruises or other markings, a review of their social support, and any physical complaints that may be indicative of trauma. The nursing diagnosis will be developed based on what is found on the assessment or considered to be most troublesome to the patient at that time. For example, it could be insomnia related to disrupted sleep from recurrent nightmares. There may also be non-physical concerns that are brought to the nurse's attention. A patient may not know how to deal with the trauma experienced and may develop maladaptive coping mechanisms. This could lead to unhealthy behaviours or patterns that the nurse should be aware of during the assessment. Behaviour such as being dismissive to

Table 10.1 Utilizing the nursing process in trauma assessments

Assessment	Considered the data collection phase, it includes gathering information about the patient's physical, spiritual, and psychosocial situation, among other data points. The nurse will use this information to better understand the patient's health status and start to develop a diagnosis
Diagnosis	Different from medical diagnoses, a nursing diagnosis is used to better understand the patient's health status and needs. The final diagnosis will drive the care plan
Planning	Often given in two separate phases, this includes planning outcomes and planning interventions. The purpose of this step is to create measurable and obtainable goals—both short and long term—for the patient while in the nurse's care. The desired outcome will drive the nursing interventions

These first three steps should be clearly documented in the patient's chart and visible to all healthcare team members.

Implementation	In this step, the nurse is carrying out what was planned above. It is critical to document all care provided and the patient's response
Evaluation	Although this may appear to be the final step, it is only final if the desired outcomes are reached. The nurse will evaluate whether their interventions were successful in treating the patient's concerns. This is a continuous process, with outcomes resolved being removed from the care plan and newly identified interventions added. It is an evolving document

ANA (2022), Wilkinson et al. (2019)

medical staff could indicate a recent trauma. Remember, the nurse will not be making a formal diagnosis of PTSD or acute stress disorder, this should be done by a mental health provider.

During the planning stage, the nurse will work with the patient to determine desired outcomes or goals for treatment. Goals should be set using the acronym SMART (specific, measurable, achievable, relevant, and time-bound) and be both long- and short-term objectives. These outcomes will drive nursing-specific interventions. Continuing with the example of insomnia, the nurse can provide education on sleep hygiene. Reinforcing that simple changes can create meaningful outcomes will lead to better results and build trust within the healthcare system. As noted in the table, these first three steps should be clearly documented in the patient's chart so all members of the treatment team can help reinforce the care delivered.

After the first three steps are completed, the nurse can then implement what was planned with the patient. If providing sleep hygiene was the intervention, the implementation could include helping the patient download a mobile application. Evaluation of the patient's outcomes and goals is a continuous process. This includes modifying interventions and reviewing what has been helpful and what has not been helpful. When a goal is met, it should be documented as such but should not be removed from the patient's chart. The possibility of a relapse of symptoms should always be considered, and it will be necessary to be able to access previous treatment plans. New symptoms may also become prevalent as others improve.

Utilizing an assessment flowchart can provide a structured, step-by-step guide to systematically evaluating trauma exposure, ensuring a comprehensive and trauma-informed approach to patient care (see Fig. 10.1). The assessment process should begin with utilizing all our senses of observing the individual, looking and listening while gathering verbal and nonverbal cues. The primary concern at this phase is being sensitive to the needs of the individual and providing a safe environment for them.

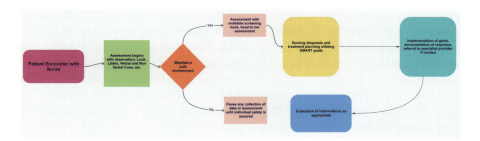

Fig. 10.1 Nursing assessment flowchart

The Screening and Diagnostic Process

Screening tools are easily accessible online and require minimal training to administer. There are fewer diagnostic tools, but they are also available to the public; however, these must be administered by mental health professionals. It is important to utilize the most appropriate tool for age, developmental level, and specialty population—such as veterans. Screening tools offer a standardized way to assess an individual's risk at any point in time and can be used to refer for a comprehensive diagnostic assessment, ensure timely treatment, and determine a plan of care. Alternatively, diagnostic tools provide trained healthcare providers with a structured set of questions to help with diagnostic clarity and understand the severity of illness. When considering a screening or diagnostic tool in practice, the nurse must make the selection based on the patient's personal history. These include a patient's age, reading and educational level, culture, language, cognition, and memory of events.

The reading and educational level of the child, caregiver, or adult can impact how questions are read or interpreted. It is important to keep in mind that it can be embarrassing to admit that one is unable to read and recommend that a patient's "preferred method of learning" be assessed as part of the intake. Everyone also experiences trauma differently, which is why the question of perceived threat is so critical. Some patients may present to a clinical setting with physical or other mental concerns and not recognize that these symptoms are manifestations of the trauma experienced. The nurse should also have the ability to provide tools in multiple languages. Trauma screening and diagnostic tools use complex wording, which can lead to misinterpretation and delayed diagnosis and referral. Finally, a patient's level of cognition and memory is another factor to consider when administering a tool. For example, has the patient experienced a traumatic brain injury (TBI), leading to impaired recall of events?

All of these factors should be considered by the nurse when determining if a screening or diagnostic tool should be self- or clinician-administered. Table 10.2 provides an outline of how to establish rapport with patients when difficult conversations or topics may be discussed. Prior to administration, depending on the setting, it is important to prepare the patient for the questions that will be asked. For example, the nurse may want to tell the patient that the screener will be discussing and asking about difficult situations. It is therapeutic to remind the patient that if at any point they wish to stop the process, they will not be judged or have care withheld. The nurse should reinforce that asking about trauma is common practice and what to expect after the process is completed.

Screening

Screening is a wide net process that can be done by any medical provider to check for any health condition before signs or symptoms emerge. Often part of the physical exam, screening tests include such things as checking blood pressure or a pap

Table 10.2 Steps to establish building rapport

1.	Setting and location	Create an environment that prioritizes patient safety and privacy. The area should be quiet, with minimal interruptions. Respect the patient's personal space. If family members are present, ask if they should be involved in the discussion
2.	Stimulation	Reduce the need for unnecessary lights, sounds and distractions. The nurse should speak softly and at a pace that promotes understanding. Keep calm if the patient is distressed
3.	Active listening	Be present and listen to what the patient is saying and may not be saying (nonverbal cues such as body language). Face the patient and use open body language. Maintain eye contact if culturally appropriate
4.	Use of silence	This allows the patient to continue to think about their responses and continue the conversation. It also shows that you are listening and processing what has been said. Try counting to 5 and if the patient has not continued, this may be your cue to begin explaining and interpreting
5.	Explaining	Discuss the process of the next steps in the evaluation and assessment. Explain the results of screening (if trained). Reinforce that some of the symptoms experienced may be related to past trauma(s)
6.	Interpretation	Restate and clarify any concepts discussed by the patient. Have them elaborate if there is still need for further interpretation
7.	Planning (follow-up/referral/monitoring)	This process includes taking all the information that has been obtained by the nurse's assessment and creating a therapeutic treatment plan. This includes appropriate referrals to mental health providers and community resources. The nurse will need to schedule follow-up appointments to allow for ongoing monitoring of symptoms

smear, with the idea to find a problem early on and be easier to treat (HHS 2021). Basic screening should also include mental health conditions, including trauma and PTSD. Unfortunately, there are a number of reasons that screening does not occur in a primary care setting. Potential barriers included patients not being sure whether to bring up their trauma, providers not knowing whether to screen, provider fear of saying the wrong thing, and the constraints and priorities of providers and patients affecting discussions of trauma (van den Berk-Clark et al. 2021).

For the adult patient population, the majority of screening tools are administered via self-report. A positive screen can be interpreted by any healthcare provider; however, nurses are often the first point of contact and spend a considerable amount of time with patients. There should be team communication of any trauma-related concerns so that appropriate resources and referrals can be put in place. Furthermore, a screen for PTSD should be part of routine care if trauma experience is disclosed.

In the paediatric population, depending on the age and developmental history of the child, the screen can be self-reported or completed by a trusted caregiver. In young children, it is recommended that a trusted adult or caregiver ask the questions, as they can be very sensitive in nature. They can read the questions in a non-threatening way that can be understood by the child. It is important to reinforce that the screen is part of routine care so as not to create any hurdles or barriers for appropriate referrals. In all cases of screening, whether adult or paediatric populations, privacy and confidentiality practices must be maintained. The only exception to this is when there may be an immediate risk of a patient harming themselves or others. Nurses should also be aware of mandatory reporting practices of abuse in their countries. In the United States, each State has their individual child and adult protective services (CPS and APS, respectively) that are run by various departments within the State. For example, it is run by the Department of Human Services in Maryland and the Department of Social Services in California.

Screening for trauma should also be completed when in contact with a patient to provide the highest level of care. Emergency department evaluations should be standard care and completed within the triage or nursing intake process. Vulnerable populations, including children, geriatrics, those with physical and cognitive impairment and developmental delays should also be screened. Screening in these population groups can be protective, as they may not be able to verbalize or understand that they are a victim of trauma or abuse. Regardless of the setting, all efforts should be made to ensure privacy and safety for the individuals being screened in the event of safety concerns and to allow for confidential disclosure.

Trauma screening should be viewed as a preventive measure that allows for early recognition and referral to a mental health specialist and treatment. A positive screen for increased risk or screening that meets the diagnostic threshold should trigger an appropriate referral for a formal diagnosis to determine appropriate treatment and plan of care. Capturing this population early will reduce the risk of negative health sequelae associated with untreated trauma scars.

Diagnosis

Appropriate diagnostic evaluations should be completed by licensed mental health specialists who are qualified to perform psychiatric and trauma assessments. While a formal diagnosis is most likely to come from a full psychiatric history and evaluation, there are tools that can be used to make a provisional diagnosis. The gold standard is the Clinician-Administered PTSD Scale for DSM-5 (CAPS-5), which was developed by the US Department of Veteran Affairs (VA). This tool provides a guideline for a structured interview that will take 40–50 min. It will identify the frequency and the intensity of PTSD symptoms, as well as symptoms commonly associated with PTSD. If there is concern for psychiatric co-morbidity, the Structured Clinical Interview for DSM (SCID) is another option (VA 2022b).

If a patient is formally diagnosed with PTSD, the nurse should be prepared for different reactions to the diagnosis. After a diagnosis, the nurse should build on the rapport developed to best understand how the patient is coping with the diagnosis. For some, it may be a relief to have an answer to the symptoms they have been experiencing. However, the range of reactions may be from disbelief or denial to embarrassment and guilt. There remains significant stigma around mental illness, and acceptance of a diagnosis and treatment can be considered a sign of weakness. Being present and an active listener can be the difference for successful treatment and recovery.

Common Screening and Diagnostic Tools Used in Practice

After the initial assessment, the nurse should then determine the appropriate tool for the setting of the evaluation and population. In primary care settings, all children, adolescents, and adults should be screened for a history of trauma. It should be considered common practice, just like asking a patient if they use tobacco or exercise. Smoking and a sedentary lifestyle can lead to poor health outcomes, and so can a history of trauma. A common tool to use for adults is the Adverse Childhood Events Questionnaire (ACE-Q). This includes ten questions that assess whether the patient experienced abuse, neglect, or household challenges as a child. Also available is the ACE International Questionnaire (ACE-IQ), which is intended for use in all countries, that asks about family dysfunction, exposure to abuse and violence, and neglect by caregivers. Up to two-thirds of the US population and 75% of those that have responded to the ACE-IQ have experienced at least one ACE, making this a common problem (CDC 2022; Pace et al. 2022). For both questionnaires, the score does not necessarily indicate the level of severity but rather indicates the risk for associated health outcomes. Regardless of the risk, all patients should be educated about the health consequences and assessed for resilience and supportive resources. Those at intermediate-to-high risk should also be linked to appropriate services and treatment (Aware 2020).

There are several other screening and diagnostic tools that are available to the public domain. Table 10.3 provides a brief overview of the ones commonly seen in both primary care and mental health practice. The US Department of Veteran Affairs (VA) has also developed several tools as many veterans (range 11–30%) will develop or experience PTSD symptoms at some point in their lifetime (VA 2022a). Regardless of the setting or population the nurse is caring for, if there is a positive screen, they will have to know the resources available for further treatment. Again, it is important to reinforce that a PTSD diagnosis can only be made by a mental health professional. However, the nurse can provide ongoing support and assessments to confirm the resolution of troublesome symptoms.

Table 10.3 Common screening and diagnostic tools for trauma

Population	Tool	Diagnosis or screening	Training	Description	Timeline	Interpretation of score
Adult	PTSD Checklist for DSM-5 (PCL-5)	Screening with provisional diagnosis	Self-report; interpreted by a clinician	A 20-item questionnaire that monitors symptoms, screens for PTSD, and can make a provisional diagnosis of PTSD Consider when unable to administer CAPS-5	Clinical judgement to monitor change and progress of treatment PCL recommendation: 5–10 point change represents reliable change, and 10–20 point change represents a clinically significant change	Three versions: (1) without Criterion A when trauma exposure is measured in another method, (2) with a brief Criterion A assessment, and (3) with the LEC-5 and extended Criterion A assessment Severity score range is from 0–80; each symptom cluster severity can be interpreted individually A provisional PTSD diagnosis can be made by treating each item rated as 2 = "Moderately" or higher as a symptom endorsed, then following the DSM-5 diagnostic rule Research has found that a score between 31 and 33 is indicative of probable PTSD https://www.ptsd.va.gov/professional/assessment/adult-sr/ptsd-checklist.asp
Adult and veteran	Clinician-Administered PTSD Scale for DSM-5 (CAPS-5) The "gold standard"	Diagnostic	Clinicians or clinical researchers; should have knowledge of PTSD diagnostic criteria	A 30-item, structured interview; to help diagnose and understand symptom severity	Three versions: (1) past week to evaluate symptoms in past week; (2) past month for current diagnostic status; and (3) worst month for lifetime PTSD	Recommend giving with the Life Events Checklist (LEC-5) A diagnosis is made when determining if a symptom is present or absent, then following the DSM-5 criteria (criterion B, C, D, E, F, and G) Weathers, F. W., Blake, D. D., Schnurr, P. P., Kaloupek, D. G., Marx, B. P., & Keane, T. M. (2015). *The Clinician-Administered PTSD Scale for DSM-5 (CAPS-5) – Past Month* [Measurement instrument]. Available from https://www.ptsd.va.gov/

10 Trauma Assessment

Adults	Brief Trauma Questionnaire (BTQ)	Screening	Self-report; qualified mental health professionals	A 10-item questionnaire; determines whether an individual has had an event that meets Criterion A using yes/no questions	Can be administered in a variety of settings to quickly screen for traumatic events	Questions 1–9 ask about events experienced, and question 10 asks about events witnessed. A response of yes in 1–9 asks additional clarifying questions about perceived or experienced threat/injury A positive score is considered when the client answers yes to "life threat or serious injury" for events 1–3 and 5–7; "life threat" for event 4; "serious injury" for event 8; or "has this ever happened to you?" for events 9 and 10 Schnurr, P., Vielhauer, M., Weathers, F., & Findler, M. (1999). The Brief Trauma Questionnaire (BTQ) [Measurement instrument]. Available from https://www.ptsd.va.gov/professional/assessment/te-measures/brief_trauma_questionnaire_btq.asp
Adults	Trauma Screening Questionnaire (TSQ)	Screening	Qualified mental health professionals and researchers; can be used by other professionals unfamiliar with the PTSD symptom clusters or diagnosis	A 10-item questionnaire to understand personal reaction to a traumatic event Yes/no answers to whether experiences occurred at least twice in the past week	Intended to be used at least 3–4 weeks post-trauma to allow for natural recovery process	Unique in that it does not require a minimum number of re-experiencing or arousal symptoms (or clusters) A report of at least six symptoms in any combination is considered to be a positive screen If a screen is positive, it is recommended by the developer to follow up with an appropriate referral and structured interview for PTSD Brewin, C. R., Rose, S., Andrews, B., Green, J., Tata, P., McEvedy, C., Turner, S., and Foa, E. B. (2002). Brief screening instrument for post-traumatic stress disorder. The British Journal of Psychiatry, 181, 158-162 https://www.ptsd.va.gov/professional/assessment/screens/tsq.asp

(continued)

Table 10.3 (continued)

Population	Tool	Diagnosis or screening	Training	Description	Timeline	Interpretation of score
Paediatrics (0–5 yrs)	Safe Environment for Every Kid Parent Questionnaire-R (SEEK PQ-R)	Screening	Intended to be completed by parents. Reviewed by PCP, SW, or other health professional	A 16-item questionnaire that assesses basic safety and then targets difficult issues Screens for psychosocial problems that can be a risk for child maltreatment	Provided to parents prior to routine visits (2, 9, and 15 months, and 2, 3, 4, and 5 years)	A screen is considered positive when "yes" is answered to the following questions: Food insecurity: either food-related question Harsh punishment: "slap or hit" question or "…child is difficult…" Major stress: "child is difficult", "more help", or "extreme stress" Depression: "feeling down" or "little interest" Intimate Partner Violence: either of the two questions Substance abuse: either question https://seekwellbeing.org/seek-materials/

Paediatric (3–17 yrs)	Child and Adolescent Trauma Screen (CATS)	Screening	Self-report for those 7–17 yrs; two caregiver versions for 3–6 yrs and 7–17 yrs	A 40-item questionnaire that measures traumatic events, DSM-5 PTSD symptoms and psychosocial functioning	Recommend using as part of a routine assessment and later for continued monitoring of symptoms; if possible, use both the self-report and caregiver screen	CATS 7–17 years: Score <15: normal, not clinically elevated Score 15–20: moderate trauma-related distress Score 21+: probably PTSD CATS 3–6 years: Score <12: normal, not clinically elevated Score 12–14: moderate trauma-related distress Score 15+: probably PTSD https://istss.org/getattachment/Clinical-Resources/Child-Trauma-Assessments/Child-and-Adolescent-Trauma-Screen-(CATS)/Clinical-Guide-for-Administering-CATS.pdf?lang=en-US https://istss.org/clinical-resources/assessing-trauma/child-and-adolescent-trauma-screen-(cats)
Paediatrics (8–17 yrs)	Trauma Symptom Checklist for Children—Screening Form (TSCC-SF)	Screening	Does not require an advanced degree or training. Recommend that the screener be trained and able to apply cut-off scores for further referral	A 20-item questionnaire that looks at general and sexual trauma and sexual concerns Screens for children at risk following a traumatic event	Administered when it is known a child or adolescent has experienced trauma	Two separate cut-off scores for those ages 8–12 years and 13–17 years Scores separately the general trauma and the sexual concerns score https://www.parinc.com/Products/Pkey/4520 Briere J., Wherry J. (2016). Development and validation of the TSCC screening form and the TSCYC screening form. Odessa, FL: Psychological Assessment Resources

(continued)

Table 10.3 (continued)

Population	Tool	Diagnosis or screening	Training	Description	Timeline	Interpretation of score
Ages 18 and older	Adverse Childhood Events—Questionnaire (ACE-Q)	Screening	Self-report	A 10-item questionnaire was used to measure trauma experiences prior to 18 years of age. Questions are categorized: abuse, neglect, and household challenges	It should be part of routine screening for all adults and completed at least once per lifetime. Consider screening on intake during PCP office visit or after rapport is built in mental health setting	Most of the general population has experienced at least one ACE. The higher the score, the more trauma a patient has experienced, and the greater the risk for negative health consequences. Felitti, V. J., Anda, R. F., Nordenberg, D., Williamson, D. F., Spitz, A. M., Edwards, V., ... Marks, J. S. (1998). Relationship of childhood abuse and household dysfunction to many of the leading causes of death in adults. The Adverse Childhood Experiences (ACE) Study. American Journal of Preventive Medicine, 14(4), 245–258 https://www.acesaware.org/wp-content/uploads/2019/12/ACE-Clinical-Workflows-Algorithms-and-ACE-Associated-Health-Conditions.pdf

| Paediatric and adolescents (ages 0–19 yrs) | Paediatric ACEs and Related Life Events Screener (PEARLS) | Screening | Self-report | There are three versions of the tool: Ages 0–11 to be completed by a caregiver, ages 12–19 to be completed by a caregiver, and adolescent self-report tool for ages 12–19 | It is recommended that children and adolescents be screened annually for risk of exposure to stress | This tool includes two parts for a total of 17 questions. Part I includes ten questions that screen for ACES, and Part II includes seven questions that screen for additional adversities or social determinants of health Part I is a score of 0–10, with a higher score indicating more ACEs experienced, rather than severity. Part II is not added to the first score and is rather used for treatment planning. Evidence suggests that exposure to other SDOH, and not just ACES, can lead to poorer health outcomes Koita, K., Long, D., Hessler, D., Benson, M., Daley, K., Bucci, M., Thakur, N., & Burke Harris, N. (2018). Development and implementation of a pediatric adverse childhood experiences (ACEs) and other determinants of health questionnaire in the pediatric medical home: A pilot study. *PloS one*, *13*(12), e0208088. https://doi.org/10.1371/journal.pone.0208088 |

For a more comprehensive list of paediatric and adolescent screens, the authors recommend this site: https://www.nctsn.org/sites/default/files/resources/complex_trauma_standardized_measures.pdf

Non-traditional Forms of Screening

Screening and diagnostic tools are not the only way to assess for trauma. Patients will present in different clinical settings, which may not always be ideal for asking multiple questions. In these cases, the nurse should be aware of alternative or non-traditional ways to identify victims of trauma.

Alternate Light Source

One such method is the use of an alternate light source (ALS), which can be used to identify bruising, specifically subtle ones that may not be noticeably visible. It has been found to be useful in improving visualization of bruises that can be observed in white or ambient light, strangulation bruises not easily seen in white light and intentionally created latent bruises (Anderson et al. 2021). There are few studies that look at the impact of using ALS to assess for potential bruises in abuse victims. One reported randomized control trial was developed to provide better insight into the use of this source for the identification of bruises (Scafide et al. 2020). Their results found that ALS wavelengths of 415 and 450 nm, when viewed through a yellow filter, detected bruising better than white light. Although this should not be considered a diagnostic tool, when used with a thorough physical examination and interview, it can help with validating a victim's trauma (Scafide et al. 2020).

Photography

Individuals who present to healthcare centres following a trauma should be assessed by an interdisciplinary team. A head-to-toe physical examination should be completed by nursing and provider staff to look for wounds or bruising that may not be visible on initial intake (i.e. triage). Many electronic health records provide the opportunity to draw on a human body outline or body part where a wound is located. However, there is also the ability to upload photographs into charts for clarity and documentation purposes. In the case of trauma or victims of assault, specially trained nurses are integral for taking clear photographs as part of the forensic medical examination. These nurses, sexual assault forensic nurse examiners, are often referred to as SANE or SAFE nurses. While there are many components to the examination, medical photography provides documentation of evidence found on a victim's body before it is collected, preserves the appearance of the injury, and can be used as a reference if needed in court or other legal proceedings (OVC 2022). Technology has further allowed for producing higher resolution images with better detail to help with detecting the age and severity of wounds or bruises. The use of a 3D surface scanner has been one new development in improved accuracy of injury documentation. It was noted in one study to have significant advantages over 2D images, such as clarity, recording of almost the full injured area, surface geometry of the area, and no need for a scale to be in the picture (Shamata and Thompson 2018).

Play and Art Therapy

The use of non-directive therapies, which do not address trauma in a direct format, allows individuals to express their experiences and emotions with a trained professional (Humble et al. 2019). Not a traditional way to screen for trauma, the use of play and art therapy can provide both children and adults the ability to communicate their histories with mental health providers. This section will not go into the details and different approaches of play and art therapy—such as child-centred play therapy (CCPT)—but rather the importance of examining this as a technique to elicit details. The unstructured format of this process relies on the professional's interpersonal skills to encourage individuals to address traumatic experiences without directly asking about the trauma (Humble et al. 2019). Using toys and a playroom that provide a non-judgemental and safe environment allows individuals, especially children, to regain trust (Parker et al. 2020). Art therapy provides a similar mode of communicating with therapists and mental health providers about previous trauma. Studies suggest that it can help aid in the recovery of or elaboration of traumatic memories (Schnitzer et al. 2021). Once memories are recovered, further screening and referral to appropriate therapies and treatments can be completed and help the patient on the path to healing.

Taking the Appropriate Next Steps

Following a positive screen or diagnosis of trauma, it is imperative for the nurse to take the appropriate next steps. The first step, as in all nursing care, is to ensure the patient is safe. This includes physical, sexual, and emotional safety; if the patient is not safe, the nurse should be aware of their role. Briefly, whenever a nurse or other interested party is made aware of an unsafe situation, it should be reported to the appropriate authorities. This includes, within the United States, child and adult protective services. Mandated reporting is reviewed in full detail in Chap. 4. Safety also includes whether a patient is a danger to themselves or others. Rates of suicide are higher in those who have experienced trauma or have a diagnosis of PTSD (Fox et al. 2021; Ásgeirsdóttir et al. 2018). Those who were exposed to violence as a child, veterans and others with a PTSD diagnosis are also at greater risk for engaging in violent behaviour. This includes physical and gun violence (Norman et al. 2020; Wamser-Nanney et al. 2019).

Once safety is evaluated, referral to appropriate resources and treatment is an important next step. The severity of psychiatric symptoms in those who have experienced trauma, regardless of the diagnosis, has been found to be greater than those who have no history of trauma. This population is also at a higher risk for relapse and poorer response to medication treatment with antidepressants (Gatov et al. 2020). Appropriate referrals can include outpatient therapy and medication management, partial hospitalization or intensive outpatient programmes, rehabilitation, or inpatient mental healthcare if warranted. The nurse should also be aware that those with a history of trauma have fewer desirable outcomes than those who have not.

This population are also more likely to have an against medical advice (AMA) discharge, lower chance of following up with a psychiatrist 30-days post discharge, increased acute care utilization in the year following discharge, and a 30% increased risk of self-harm in the following year (Gatov et al. 2020).

Case: New-Onset Stomach Pain

Child: Antonio
Age: 11
Setting: School nurse's office

Current presentation: This is Antonio's fourth presentation to the school nurse in the past month. During the first three visits, he was encouraged to go by the cafeteria staff, as he often eats his full tray of food. When he stopped eating as much, they became concerned. He did not eat his lunch three times, citing stomach pain, and they referred him to the school nurse. The findings by the school nurse were benign and attributed the pains to the quality of the meals in the cafeteria. During these visits, Antonio would stay until the end of the lunch period, talking with the nurse if she was not busy. He began to trust her and feel safe and comfortable in the office.

During his fourth visit, Antonio not only comes in with stomach pain but also has bruising on his lower arms. The nurse questions the bruising, which he initially states is from football practice, but he becomes tearful. He begins to share with the nurse about his mother's new boyfriend, John, who moved into the apartment about two months ago. Initially, he was excited to have a male figure back in his life after the passing of his biological father four years prior. However, as John became more comfortable with the new living arrangements, Antonio noticed a change in his behaviour and demeanour. John would come home from work late more often, usually under the influence of alcohol. John then started to become more argumentative with his mother, blaming her for food being cooked improperly, the house being dirty, and how well the kids were behaving. Many times, John would strike his mother in front of him and his younger brother. John had never hit him, but the night prior to this office visit, Antonio had attempted to get between his mother and John. This resulted in a physical confrontation between the two. This is all Antonio will confide in me, and he does not go into further detail about the confrontation. Antonio asks the nurse to keep this between the two of them and asks her to promise him she will not tell anyone. He states that he is worried that John might "do something bad" to him and his family if she says something.

Reflection Questions

1. What is the role of the school nurse in reporting suspected abuse? Putting yourself in the position of the nurse, how would you tell Antonio about your next steps while still maintaining the therapeutic relationship created?

2. What are the nurse's top priorities in treating Antonio?
3. Reflecting on the ACEs questionnaire, what has Antonio experienced at this point in his life?

Summary

Nurses are in a unique position to be one of the initial members of a treatment team to interact with a patient. They have the opportunity to ask about personal and social history, which should include trauma, perform safety assessments, and review screening and diagnostic results. Utilizing the four Rs approach developed by SAMHSA, the nurse is provided with the ability to be more inclusive in their trauma assessments. This involves realizing the impact of trauma and recovery options, recognizing the signs and symptoms in all interested parties, responding with knowledge about trauma, and resisting re-traumatization (SAMHSA 2014).

This chapter also reviewed the use of screening tools to assess an individual's risk and need for referral to receive a more comprehensive diagnostic assessment. Diagnostic tools are also available to trained healthcare providers, which can lead to diagnostic clarity and illness severity. When selecting the appropriate tool, the nurse should always consider the patient's individual characteristics for the most accurate score interpretation. Simultaneously, the nursing process is being utilized for the best patient outcomes. It has been well documented that patients with trauma histories have poorer outcomes than those without. Nurses are given the unique opportunity to address these barriers and improve the aftermath experienced simply by recognizing and referring to treatment.

Discussion Question

A 16-year-old student was recently involved in a motor vehicle accident with two fatalities. How would you use the nursing process to create a trauma-informed nursing treatment plan? Consider using the template provided to organize your thoughts.

Population	Tool
Assessment	
Diagnosis	
Planning outcomes	
Planning interventions	
Implementation	
Evaluation	
Follow-up and modifications	

Concepts

ACES
Screening tools vs provisional diagnosis
Cut-off points
Diagnostic tools
Gold standard

References

ANA (2022) The nursing process. https://www.nursingworld.org/practice-policy/workforce/what-is-nursing/the-nursing-process/

Anderson JC, Pollitt EN, Schildbach C, MacDonald R, Rose L, Sheridan DJ (2021) Alternate light source findings of common topical cosmetics and three removal methods. J Forensic Nurs 17(1):14–23. https://doi.org/10.1097/jfn.0000000000000300

Ásgeirsdóttir HG, Valdimarsdóttir UA, Þorsteinsdóttir ÞK, Lund SH, Tomasson G, Nyberg U et al (2018) The association between different traumatic life events and suicidality. Eur J Psychotraumatol 9(1):1510279. https://doi.org/10.1080/20008198.2018.1510279

Aware A (2020) ACE screening clinical workflows, ACEs and toxic stress risk assessment algorithm, and ACE-associated health conditions: for pediatrics and adults. https://www.acesaware.org/wp-content/uploads/2019/12/ACE-Clinical-Workflows-Algorithms-and-ACE-Associated-Health-Conditions.pdf

CDC (2022) Fast facts: preventing adverse childhood experiences. https://www.cdc.gov/violenceprevention/aces/fastfact.html

Fox V, Dalman C, Dal H, Hollander AC, Kirkbride JB, Pitman A (2021) Suicide risk in people with post-traumatic stress disorder: a cohort study of 3.1 million people in Sweden. J Affect Disord 279:609–616. https://doi.org/10.1016/j.jad.2020.10.009

Gatov E, Koziel N, Kurdyak P, Saunders NR, Chiu M, Lebenbaum M et al (2020) Discharge and post-discharge outcomes of psychiatric inpatients with a lifetime history of exposure to interpersonal trauma: a population-based study. Gen Hosp Psychiatry 65:82–90. https://doi.org/10.1016/j.genhosppsych.2020.05.015

HHS (2021) Get screened. U.S. Department of Health and Human Services. https://health.gov/myhealthfinder/doctor-visits/screening-tests/get-screened

Humble JJ, Summers NL, Villarreal V, Styck KM, Sullivan JR, Hechler JM, Warren BS (2019) Child-centered play therapy for youths who have experienced trauma: a systematic literature review. J Child Adolesc Trauma 12(3):365–375. https://doi.org/10.1007/s40653-018-0235-7

Norman S, Elbogen EB, Schnurr PP (2020) Research findings on PTSD and violence. https://www.ptsd.va.gov/professional/treat/cooccurring/research_violence.asp

OVC (2022) SANE program development and operation guide: photo documentation. Office for Victims of Crime. https://www.ovcttac.gov/saneguide/identifying-essential-components-of-a-sane-program/photo-documentation/

Pace CS, Muzi S, Rogier G, Meinero LL, Marcenaro S (2022) The adverse childhood experiences – international questionnaire (ACE-IQ) in community samples around the world: a systematic review (part I). Child Abuse Negl 129:105640. https://doi.org/10.1016/j.chiabu.2022.105640

Parker MM, Hergenrather KC, Smelser QK, Kelly C (2020) Exploring child-centered play therapy and trauma: A systematic review of literature. International journal of play. Therapy 30:2

SAMHSA (2014) SAMHSA's concept of trauma and guidance for a trauma-informed approach. Retrieved from https://ncsacw.acf.hhs.gov/userfiles/files/SAMHSA_Trauma.pdf

Scafide KN, Sheridan DJ, Downing NR, Hayat MJ (2020) Detection of inflicted bruises by alternate light: results of a randomized controlled trial. J Forensic Sci 65(4):1191–1198. https://doi.org/10.1111/1556-4029.14294

Schnitzer G, Holttum S, Huet V (2021) A systematic literature review of the impact of art therapy upon post-traumatic stress disorder. Int J Art Ther 26(4):147–160. https://doi.org/10.1080/17454832.2021.1910719

Shamata A, Thompson T (2018) Documentation and analysis of traumatic injuries in clinical forensic medicine involving structured light three-dimensional surface scanning versus photography. J Forensic Leg Med 58:93–100. https://doi.org/10.1016/j.jflm.2018.05.004

VA (2022a) How common is PTSD in veterans. https://www.ptsd.va.gov/understand/common/common_veterans.asp

VA (2022b) How is PTSD assessed? https://www.ptsd.va.gov/understand/common/common_veterans.asp

van den Berk-Clark C, Gallamore R, Barnes J, Oberle A, Meyer D, Schneider FD (2021) Identifying and overcoming barriers to trauma screening in the primary care setting. Fam Syst Health 39(2):177–187. https://doi.org/10.1037/fsh0000593

Wamser-Nanney R, Nanney JT, Conrad E, Constans JI (2019) Childhood trauma exposure and gun violence risk factors among victims of gun violence. Psychol Trauma 11(1):99–106. https://doi.org/10.1037/tra0000410

Wilkinson JM, Treas LS, Smith MH, Barnett KL (2019) Davis advantage for fundamentals of nursing (2 volume set). F. A. Davis Company

Trauma: Biological Outcomes

11

Tamar Rodney

Objectives
- Analyse brain and body changes from trauma, focusing on stress hormones and physiological responses
- Explore trauma's effects on biological factors like genetics and inflammation and their long-term health impact

Introduction

Trauma, an experience that disrupts an individual's sense of stability and security, poses complex challenges for health professionals. Understanding the biological underpinnings of trauma is essential, as it significantly impacts health and well-being. Recent advancements in neuroscience have highlighted how trauma impacts brain structure and function (Giotakos 2020; Singh et al. 2021). Understanding these n eurobiological shifts is crucial, as they offer insights into potential therapeutic interventions.

Trauma can trigger a cascade of neurobiological changes, affecting brain function, hormone regulation, and overall physiology. These alterations not only influence immediate responses but can also have lasting effects, shaping emotional regulation, cognitive processes, and physical health over time (Services 2016). By exploring the intricate connections between trauma and biological factors, including genetics and inflammation, we can gain deeper insights into the mechanisms of trauma and develop more effective interventions for those affected. This knowledge is vital for healthcare professionals aiming to provide holistic and informed care to individuals with trauma histories.

T. Rodney (✉)
Johns Hopkins University School of Nursing, Baltimore, MD, USA
e-mail: trodney1@jhu.edu

© The Author(s), under exclusive license to Springer Nature Switzerland AG 2025
T. Rodney (ed.), *Trauma Informed Care*,
https://doi.org/10.1007/978-3-031-87526-7_11

Neurobiological Changes

Trauma induces significant neurobiological changes that affect both brain structure and function. Key areas of the brain, such as the amygdala, hippocampus, and prefrontal cortex, undergo alterations in response to traumatic experiences (Bremner and Wittbrodt 2020; Giotakos 2020). The amygdala, responsible for processing emotions and threats, may become hyperactive, leading to heightened anxiety and fear responses (Alexandra Kredlow et al. 2022). In contrast, the hippocampus, which is crucial for memory formation and emotional regulation, can shrink in size due to chronic stress, impairing the ability to process memories accurately (Kim et al. 2015). The prefrontal cortex, associated with decision-making and impulse control, may show reduced activity, resulting in difficulties with emotional regulation and increased impulsivity (Friedman and Robbins 2022).

Trauma also affects the levels of stress hormones like cortisol and adrenaline. Cortisol, known as the "stress hormone", can become chronically elevated, disrupting the body's normal stress response and impacting the immune system, metabolism, and mood regulation. Similarly, adrenaline, which is crucial for the immediate "fight-or-flight" response, may remain dysregulated, leading to persistent anxiety and hyperarousal. While acute trauma can trigger a rapid increase in these hormones to prepare the body for immediate action, prolonged exposure can interfere with normal physiological processes, resulting in chronic health issues (Noushad et al. 2021). Additionally, neurotransmitter systems such as serotonin and dopamine can be affected. A depletion of serotonin, which helps stabilize mood, may contribute to mood disorders and depression (Jauhar et al. 2023; Troubat et al. 2021). Changes in dopamine levels, linked to reward and motivation, can impact an individual's ability to feel pleasure, leading to apathy or anhedonia. Disruptions in these neurotransmitter systems can exacerbate various psychological issues, including depression and anxiety disorders, making recovery even more challenging (Baik 2020).

Physiological Responses to Trauma

The physiological responses to trauma are often characterized by the activation of the fight-or-flight response, which prepares the body to react to perceived threats. This response involves a complex interplay of neural and hormonal changes that enhance survival in dangerous situations. While this response can be beneficial in the short term, prolonged activation can lead to long-term physiological changes. For example, chronic stress can result in elevated heart rates and blood pressure, increasing the risk of cardiovascular diseases (Kivimäki and Steptoe 2018; Osborne et al. 2020). Furthermore, the immune system can become dysregulated, leading to increased susceptibility to infections and other health issues (Quiros-Roldan et al. 2024). In addition to cardiovascular effects, trauma can also influence metabolic processes. Individuals with a history of trauma may experience changes in appetite and weight regulation, contributing to obesity or other metabolic disorders

(Dakanalis et al. 2023; Farr et al. 2014). Understanding these physiological changes is crucial for developing comprehensive treatment strategies that address both the mental and physical health needs of trauma-affected individuals (Chu et al. 2024).

Genetic and Epigenetic Factors

Genetic and epigenetic factors also play a critical role in the biological basis of trauma (Heinzelmann and Gill 2013; Thumfart et al. 2022). Some individuals may have genetic predispositions that influence their response to traumatic events, affecting their vulnerability to developing post-traumatic stress disorder (PTSD) (Al Jowf et al. 2021; Cao-Lei et al. 2022; Chou et al. 2024) or other mental health issues (Thumfart et al. 2022). Research has identified specific genetic markers associated with heightened sensitivity to stress and trauma, suggesting that biology can significantly impact an individual's experience of trauma (Yehuda and Lehrner 2018). Epigenetic changes, which involve modifications in gene expression without altering the underlying DNA sequence, can occur as a result of trauma exposure. These changes can affect how individuals respond to stress throughout their lives and may even be passed down through generations, highlighting the intergenerational transmission of trauma effects. Understanding these genetic and epigenetic mechanisms is vital for developing targeted interventions that consider an individual's biological makeup.

Inflammatory Responses

Inflammatory responses are another key aspect of the biological impact of trauma. Research has shown a strong link between trauma and chronic inflammation, which can have wide-ranging effects on physical health (Hori and Kim 2019). Trauma exposure can trigger an inflammatory response in the body, leading to elevated levels of pro-inflammatory cytokines (Devoto et al. 2017; Rodney et al. 2020). Chronic inflammation has been associated with various health problems, including autoimmune disorders, cardiovascular disease, and even certain cancers (Gill et al. 2018). This connection between trauma and inflammation underscores the importance of addressing the physiological aspects of trauma in treatment (Rodney et al. 2018). Interventions that focus on reducing inflammation, such as dietary changes, exercise, and stress-reduction techniques, can be beneficial in improving overall health outcomes for trauma-affected individuals.

Trauma and Long-Term Health Effects

The long-term health effects of trauma are profound and multifaceted. Individuals with trauma histories are at an increased risk for chronic diseases, including diabetes, heart disease, and various mental health conditions, such as PTSD and depression (Hoerster et al. 2019). These connections highlight the need for a comprehensive understanding of how trauma impacts both mental and physical health over time. Moreover, the cumulative effects of trauma can lead to a cycle of health disparities, as individuals who have experienced trauma may face barriers to accessing appropriate healthcare (Ranjbar et al. 2020). This necessitates an integrated approach that addresses the full spectrum of trauma's impact on health, ensuring that individuals receive the support they need (Ranjbar et al. 2020; Services 2016).

Implications for Treatment and Intervention

Understanding the biological basis of trauma has significant implications for treatment and intervention (Services 2016). A biological perspective enhances our comprehension of the mechanisms behind trauma responses, informing the development of effective care strategies. Integrating trauma-informed care approaches, which emphasize safety, empowerment, and collaboration, can help healthcare professionals provide more holistic support for trauma-affected individuals. Moreover, incorporating evidence-based interventions that target both the psychological and physiological aspects of trauma is essential. Mindfulness practices, cognitive-behavioural therapies, and lifestyle modifications can be instrumental in promoting resilience and recovery. By addressing the interconnectedness of trauma's biological and psychological effects, we can foster more effective and compassionate care (Aarts et al. 2024) (Table 11.1).

Table 11.1 Trauma outcomes

Trauma outcomes	Key points
Neurobiological changes	Brain Areas: Amygdala (hyperactivity leads to anxiety), Hippocampus (shrinks, affecting memory), Prefrontal Cortex (reduced activity, affecting decision-making).
	Hormonal Changes: Chronic elevation of cortisol (affects stress response, immune system) and dysregulated adrenaline (leads to anxiety).
	Neurotransmitter Effects: Decreased serotonin (linked to mood disorders), altered dopamine (affects pleasure and motivation).
Physiological responses	Fight-or-Flight Activation: Short-term benefits but long-term physiological changes (elevated heart rate, blood pressure).
	Health Risks: Increased risk of cardiovascular diseases and metabolic disorders (obesity, appetite changes).
Genetic & epigenetic factors	Genetic predispositions can influence trauma response and vulnerability to PTSD.
	Epigenetic changes affect stress response and may be passed to future generations.
Inflammatory responses	Trauma can trigger chronic inflammation (elevated pro-inflammatory cytokines).
	Linked to autoimmune disorders, cardiovascular disease, and certain cancers.

Conclusion

Exploring the biological basis of trauma provides vital insights into the mechanisms underlying its impact on health and well-being. This knowledge not only enhances our understanding of trauma's effects but also informs the development of trauma-informed care approaches. Continued research in this area is essential for improving outcomes and providing comprehensive support for individuals navigating the complex landscape of trauma recovery. By bridging the gap between biological understanding and clinical practice, we can better address the needs of those affected by trauma and promote healing on multiple levels.

References

Aarts I, Thorsen AL, Vriend C, Planting C, van den Heuvel OA, Thomaes K (2024) Effects of psychotherapy on brain activation during negative emotional processing in patients with posttraumatic stress disorder: a systematic review and meta-analysis. Brain Imaging Behav 18(2):444–455. https://doi.org/10.1007/s11682-023-00831-0

Al Jowf GI, Snijders C, Rutten BPF, de Nijs L, Eijssen LMT (2021) The molecular biology of susceptibility to post-traumatic stress disorder: highlights of epigenetics and epigenomics. Int J Mol Sci 22(19). https://doi.org/10.3390/ijms221910743

Alexandra Kredlow M, Fenster RJ, Laurent ES, Ressler KJ, Phelps EA (2022) Prefrontal cortex, amygdala, and threat processing: implications for PTSD. Neuropsychopharmacology 47(1):247–259. https://doi.org/10.1038/s41386-021-01155-7

Baik JH (2020) Stress and the dopaminergic reward system. Exp Mol Med 52(12):1879–1890. https://doi.org/10.1038/s12276-020-00532-4

Bremner JD, Wittbrodt MT (2020) Stress, the brain, and trauma spectrum disorders. Int Rev Neurobiol 152:1–22. https://doi.org/10.1016/bs.irn.2020.01.004

Cao-Lei L, Saumier D, Fortin J, Brunet A (2022) A narrative review of the epigenetics of post-traumatic stress disorder and post-traumatic stress disorder treatment. Front Psych 13:857087. https://doi.org/10.3389/fpsyt.2022.857087

Chou PC, Huang YC, Yu S (2024) Mechanisms of epigenetic inheritance in post-traumatic stress disorder. Life (Basel) 14(1). https://doi.org/10.3390/life14010098

Chu B, Marwaha K, Sanvictores T, Awosika AO, Ayers D (2024) Physiology, stress reaction. In: StatPearls. StatPearls Publishing

Dakanalis A, Mentzelou M, Papadopoulou SK, Papandreou D, Spanoudaki M, Vasios GK et al (2023) The association of emotional eating with overweight/obesity, depression, anxiety/stress, and dietary patterns: a review of the current clinical evidence. Nutrients 15(5). https://doi.org/10.3390/nu15051173

Devoto C, Arcurio L, Fetta J, Ley M, Rodney T, Kanefsky R, Gill J (2017) Inflammation relates to chronic behavioral and neurological symptoms in military personnel with traumatic brain injuries. Cell Transplant 26(7):1169–1177. https://doi.org/10.1177/0963689717714098

Farr OM, Sloan DM, Keane TM, Mantzoros CS (2014) Stress- and PTSD-associated obesity and metabolic dysfunction: a growing problem requiring further research and novel treatments. Metabolism 63(12):1463–1468. https://doi.org/10.1016/j.metabol.2014.08.009

Friedman NP, Robbins TW (2022) The role of prefrontal cortex in cognitive control and executive function. Neuropsychopharmacology 47(1):72–89. https://doi.org/10.1038/s41386-021-01132-0

Gill J, Mustapic M, Diaz-Arrastia R, Lange R, Gulyani S, Diehl T et al (2018) Higher exosomal tau, amyloid-beta 42 and IL-10 are associated with mild TBIs and chronic symptoms in military personnel. Brain Inj 32(10):1277–1284. https://doi.org/10.1080/02699052.2018.1471738

Giotakos O (2020) Neurobiology of emotional trauma. Psychiatriki 31(2):162–171. https://doi.org/10.22365/jpsych.2020.312.162

Heinzelmann M, Gill J (2013) Epigenetic mechanisms shape the biological response to trauma and risk for PTSD: a critical review. Nurs Res Pract 2013:417010. https://doi.org/10.1155/2013/417010

Hoerster KD, Campbell S, Dolan M, Stappenbeck CA, Yard S, Simpson T, Nelson KM (2019) PTSD is associated with poor health behavior and greater Body Mass Index through depression, increasing cardiovascular disease and diabetes risk among U.S. veterans. Prev Med Rep 15:100930. https://doi.org/10.1016/j.pmedr.2019.100930

Hori H, Kim Y (2019) Inflammation and post-traumatic stress disorder. Psychiatry Clin Neurosci 73(4):143–153. https://doi.org/10.1111/pcn.12820

Jauhar S, Cowen PJ, Browning M (2023) Fifty years on: serotonin and depression. J Psychopharmacol 37(3):237–241. https://doi.org/10.1177/02698811231161813

Kim EJ, Pellman B, Kim JJ (2015) Stress effects on the hippocampus: a critical review. Learn Mem 22(9):411–416. https://doi.org/10.1101/lm.037291.114

Kivimäki M, Steptoe A (2018) Effects of stress on the development and progression of cardiovascular disease. Nat Rev Cardiol 15(4):215–229. https://doi.org/10.1038/nrcardio.2017.189

Noushad S, Ahmed S, Ansari B, Mustafa UH, Saleem Y, Hazrat H (2021) Physiological biomarkers of chronic stress: a systematic review. Int J Health Sci (Qassim) 15(5):46–59

Osborne MT, Shin LM, Mehta NN, Pitman RK, Fayad ZA, Tawakol A (2020) Disentangling the links between psychosocial stress and cardiovascular disease. Circ Cardiovasc Imaging 13(8):e010931. https://doi.org/10.1161/circimaging.120.010931

Quiros-Roldan E, Sottini A, Natali PG, Imberti L (2024) The impact of immune system aging on infectious diseases. Microorganisms 12(4). https://doi.org/10.3390/microorganisms12040775

Ranjbar N, Erb M, Mohammad O, Moreno FA (2020) Trauma-informed care and cultural humility in the mental health care of people from minoritized communities. Focus (Am Psychiatr Publ) 18(1):8–15. https://doi.org/10.1176/appi.focus.20190027

Rodney T, Osier N, Gill J (2018) Pro- and anti-inflammatory biomarkers and traumatic brain injury outcomes: a review. Cytokine 110:248–256. https://doi.org/10.1016/j.cyto.2018.01.012

Rodney T, Taylor P, Dunbar K, Perrin N, Lai C, Roy M, Gill J (2020) High IL-6 in military personnel relates to multiple traumatic brain injuries and post-traumatic stress disorder. Behav Brain Res 392:112715. https://doi.org/10.1016/j.bbr.2020.112715

Services, U. S. D. H. H (2016) A treatment improvement protocol – trauma-informed care in behavioral health services – tip 57. Lulu.com

Singh J, Prakash J, Yadav P, Bharti A, Chatterjee K (2021) Complex psychological trauma. Ind Psychiatry J 30(Suppl 1):S305–s307. https://doi.org/10.4103/0972-6748.328837

Thumfart KM, Jawaid A, Bright K, Flachsmann M, Mansuy IM (2022) Epigenetics of childhood trauma: long term sequelae and potential for treatment. Neurosci Biobehav Rev 132:1049–1066. https://doi.org/10.1016/j.neubiorev.2021.10.042

Troubat R, Barone P, Leman S, Desmidt T, Cressant A, Atanasova B et al (2021) Neuroinflammation and depression: a review. Eur J Neurosci 53(1):151–171. https://doi.org/10.1111/ejn.14720

Yehuda R, Lehrner A (2018) Intergenerational transmission of trauma effects: putative role of epigenetic mechanisms. World Psychiatry 17(3):243–257. https://doi.org/10.1002/wps.20568

Trauma and Resilience

12

Tamar Rodney , Pearl Ed Cuevas, Thitipong Tankampuan, Rajesh Kumar, Veroina Deslandes, Chitchanok Benjasirisan, and Suratsawadee Kruahong

Objectives
- Explore coping with trauma using the Society-to-Cells Theoretical Framework.
- Identify various coping strategies and support systems for individual, family, and community exposed to traumatic events or situations across the lifespan.

Introduction

Recovery from trauma is a process that relies on both individual resilience and supportive environments, drawing on personal strength and external support systems. Using a Society-to-Cells Theoretical Framework provides a holistic view of trauma recovery, emphasizing how layers of support—societal, community, family, and individual—contribute to healing. Cultural attitudes towards mental health often

---

T. Rodney · C. Benjasirisan · S. Kruahong
Johns Hopkins University School of Nursing, Baltimore, MD, USA
e-mail: trodney1@jhu.edu; cbenjas1@jhmi.edu; skruaho1@jhmi.edu

P. E. Cuevas
Centro Escolar University Manila, Manila, Philippines

T. Tankampuan
Mahidol University Faculty of Nursing, Bangkok, Thailand
e-mail: thitipong.tan@mahidol.ac.th

R. Kumar (✉)
All India Institute of Medical Sciences, Rishikesh, Uttarakhand, India
e-mail: rajesh.nur@aiimsrishikesh.edu.in

V. Deslandes
University of the West Indies-Mona, Kingston, Jamaica
e-mail: veroina.deslandes@uwimona.edu.jm

© The Author(s), under exclusive license to Springer Nature Switzerland AG 2025
T. Rodney (ed.), *Trauma Informed Care*,
https://doi.org/10.1007/978-3-031-87526-7_12

impact individuals' willingness to seek help, as stigma and trust in non-professional support systems frequently shape their choices. Many people turn to family, clergy, or community resources before seeking professional mental health services, with some preferring informal help as a first step toward recovery. Acknowledging these preferences is essential to fostering trauma recovery in ways that are both effective and culturally sensitive, promoting resilience across diverse backgrounds and life stages.

Explore Trauma as Experienced in Different Regions in the World

Caribbean

The recovery process from a traumatic experience, whether a personal tragedy or a global disaster, will take an emotional toll on the individual, family, community, or nation. The psychological impact of the trauma on the person will depend on how he or she perceives the degree of trauma or experiences trauma and what adaptive measures and protective factors can be utilized in coping with the event or situation for a better outcome.

Considering the high rate of violence being experienced by the children, youth, and women in Latin America and the Caribbean (LAC). One way to address the perennial problem is to approach it from a multidisciplinary and multisectoral point of view, to bring about organizational changes in the behavioural health sector, juvenile justice system, educational and economic sectors, and how to build resilience in the populace. There is evidence that reveals information about the person being resilient to various types of traumas during their lifetime. Literature speaks about the protective factors that act as a buffer to the person coping with adversities. For example, the evidence-based interventions for infants speak to the dyadic therapies of child–parent psychotherapy (CPP), parent–child interaction therapy (PCIT), and trauma-focused cognitive behaviour therapy (TF-CBT) (Earls 2018). During the parent–child attachment, they are able to form a strong bond which serves as a source of trust and self-confidence.

The family is the first social agent that is responsible for providing the basic necessities and skills for the child to develop and be able to cope with adversity throughout the life span. Therefore, corporal punishment should be prohibited as a form of discipline, whether at home or in school. Children who are exposed to violence are likely to become victims or perpetrators of violence in later life, which is eventually implicated in the high incidence of intimate partner violence currently seen in LAC (WHO 2020a, b; Guedes 2018). Strategies to build resilience within a child can be developed through positive parenting, providing the basic necessities (shelter, food, clothing), completing secondary school education, and being gainfully employed.

The World Health Organization realizes the importance of the prevention of violence against children and collaborates with other organizations to develop and endorse an evidence-based technical package called INSPIRE—strategies intended for ending violence against children, which have been proven to produce favourable results in other regions and can be adapted to the Latin America and the Caribbean region.

1. The implementation and enforcement of laws (restricting access to alcohol and firearms)
2. Norms and values change (altering norms that condone the sexual abuse of girls or aggressive behaviour)
3. Safe environments
4. Parental and caregiver support
5. Income and economic strengthening
6. Education and life skills
7. Response services provision (appropriate psychological care)

Citizens of Latin America and the Caribbean regions are known to exhibit various coping strategies in the advent of adversities such as high rate of crime and violence, high homicide rates, increased road fatalities due to motor vehicle accidents that result in the sudden death of loved ones, and increased intimate partner violence against women and girls. In addition, those people who live in the Caribbean must be contented with the unpredictability of the annual hurricane season, which can result in widespread disaster and destruction of life and property (Maharaj, et al. 2024).

The high prevalence of violence against women and girls in the LAC permeates women of all ages, educational backgrounds, and socioeconomic statuses; in many instances, the survivor does not seek help from an institution or agency but instead turns to friends, family, and neighbours for support as means of coping with the problems (Haarr 2020).

Other ways of building resilience against challenges include the enhancement of psychosocial support, psychological intervention for survivors of intimate partner violence (IPV) combined with economic and social empowerment, and community involvement to change unequal gender norms; school programmes that enhance safety in school, reduce/eliminate harsh punishment including programme to challenge gender stereotypes, and promote relationships based on equality and consent play a crucial role. Group-based participatory education with women and men can also generate critical reflections about unequal gender power relationships (Earls 2018; SAMHSA 2014).

South and South East Asia

Thailand

Coping Strategies and Resilience Across the Lifespan
Coping strategies and resilience across cultures are significantly shaped by cultural norms, social dynamics, and individual beliefs. In Thailand, resilience and coping behaviours vary widely across different life stages and are deeply influenced by

cultural traditions, spiritual beliefs, and environmental factors (Szanton and Gill 2010). The "society-to-cell" framework emphasizes the cumulative impact of external (society, community, family) and internal (physiological, genetic) factors that jointly contribute to resilience.

Children and Adolescents

For children and adolescents, resilience is largely built within the family and community environment, which is especially vital when facing trauma or disaster. Thai studies reveal that children with chronic illness or who experience natural disasters demonstrate greater resilience when supported by strong family structures, even in stigmatized situations (Malee et al. 2019). During the 2004 tsunami and 2011 floods, many Thai youths struggled with poor psychological outcomes, but children with family and friend support exhibited stronger coping behaviours. In cases of school bullying or cyberbullying, adolescents may initially adopt avoidant strategies but are increasingly seeking help from friends, family, or teachers. However, in digital spaces, many still avoid conflict, likely due to concerns that adults may not understand the online environment or intervene effectively (Sittichai and Smith 2018). Strengthening these support networks, particularly within family and school, can help youth navigate trauma more effectively and build resilience.

Adults

Adult resilience often centres on handling multiple life stressors, such as intimate partner violence (IPV), job pressures, or health issues. In Thai culture, where self-reliance and family loyalty are valued, individuals often keep experiences of IPV or personal hardship private, with women, in particular, feeling societal pressure to manage difficulties independently. Spirituality and religious practices provide a key coping mechanism, particularly among Buddhists, who may use practices like meditation or offerings to monks as tools to promote mental well-being and acceptance of hardships (Kudva et al. 2020). Self-reliance and spiritual beliefs, while fostering personal strength, may also deter individuals from seeking formal mental health support, which remains stigmatized and relatively under-resourced in Thai society.

Older Adults

The ageing population in Thailand, now a full-fledged ageing society, faces unique challenges. Thai elders commonly employ strategies rooted in cultural and spiritual beliefs, like continuing to work, expressing "Jai-Yai" (courage), and embracing acceptance of hardships ("Plong" and "Taam-Jai"). Family is central to elder care; however, shifts towards nuclear family structures and urban migration have reduced close-knit support, leaving some elders feeling disconnected (Manasatchakun et al. 2018). Thai elders often look to cultural practices or spiritual guidance, such as consulting monks or relying on community customs, for strength in adversity. The shift in family dynamics calls for an increased focus on community-based programmes that offer social support and foster resilience.

Table 12.1 Coping strategies across lifespan in Thailand

Country		Children and adolescents	Adults	Older adults
Thailand	Coping strategies	Seeking help and expressing worries to friends and trusted adults Passive strategies: avoidance and ignoring	Keeping adverse experiences silent Self-reliance Seeking emotional support by talking with family, healthcare providers, social services, and religion Religion activities	Keep doing a job and earning a living Having courage and toughness to withstand adverse conditions Expressing difficulty Connecting with people, beliefs, and customs
	Main supportive system	Caregiver, depending on the relationship, socioeconomic status, level of education Thrust adults: family and teacher Peers	One-Stop Crisis Centres from the Thai government and non-government organizations Emotional support from family, healthcare providers, social services, and religion	Friends Siblings Family members Supportive system from personal belief: fortune teller or Monk

In summary, resilience and coping mechanisms in Thailand reflect a strong cultural emphasis on family and community support, self-reliance, and spiritual guidance. Across the lifespan, the integration of familial, social, and cultural factors remains vital to fostering resilience, though shifts in societal structures present ongoing challenges for sustaining this support, especially for the elderly (see Table 12.1).

Strengthening Resilience Through the Support System in Thailand

Despite a strong emphasis on family and community support among Thai individuals, optimizing coping and resilience requires multilevel contributions from various stakeholders. The following suggestions aim to strengthen resilience within Thailand's support system:

1. *Effective Leadership*
    Building effective leadership at the national, local, and micro-community levels is crucial. Leaders, such as district chiefs, village headmen, and religious figures, should communicate the benefits of the health system to enhance com-

munity resilience and foster trust. They must prepare for challenges by establishing emergency management plans with diverse stakeholders and ensuring transparent communication during crises. This approach can reduce trauma and facilitate community recovery.

2. *Organizational Learning Culture*

    Promoting a learning culture within organizations can enhance crisis response. Communities affected by recurrent flooding learn to monitor warning signs and adapt, yet solutions often originate at the household level. Encouraging organizations to adopt lessons from past incidents can better prepare communities and minimize losses during disasters.

3. *Access to Reliable Information*

    Ensuring a reliable flow of information is vital for decision-making during crises. Although urban areas have internet access, many rural residents lack timely updates about disasters. Improving infrastructure to connect all Thai citizens to reliable information, along with investing in surveillance systems, can help predict and mitigate the effects of future crises.

4. *Stability of Health System Funding*

    Maintaining stable funding for healthcare is essential, especially during health-related crises like the COVID-19 pandemic. Increased funding and a flexible financing plan can bolster the healthcare system's ability to respond to emergencies effectively. The pandemic highlighted the need for better financial management to sustain health coverage, even during challenging times.

5. *Equitable Resource Distribution*

    Ensuring that healthcare resources, both human and physical, are distributed appropriately is crucial. Currently, urban areas receive more attention, leaving rural populations underserved. Expanding quality resources to these areas can enhance resilience and prevent negative outcomes.

6. *Support from Healthcare Providers*

    Enhancing mental, physical, and social health through healthcare providers can improve coping mechanisms among Thai individuals. Since many underutilize healthcare services or do not recognize the health implications of trauma, nurses can raise awareness and provide assessments during patient encounters. Additionally, facilitating cognitive behavioural therapy and peer support groups can help individuals share strategies and build resilience.

7. *Trauma-Informed Care*

    Implementing trauma-informed care can support recovery for individuals with traumatic experiences. This approach fosters safety, dignity, and control, encouraging individuals to share their experiences with trusted providers, ultimately aiding their recovery process.

8. *Research on Resilience and Trauma*

    Conducting research focused on resilience, coping skills, and trauma exposure in the Thai context will deepen understanding and enhance care approaches. Research tailored to the unique behaviours and beliefs of the Thai population can inform effective interventions and raise awareness of trauma's impact, helping prevent re-traumatization in healthcare settings.

Philippines and Japan

In the Philippines, analyses of secondary datasets (Rivera et al. 2018) show that most individuals injured from trauma are young and male. There is no notable seasonality; however, more reported injuries occur on Sundays and during the daytime. The top causes of injuries in the Philippines are transport injuries and falls, leading to significant implications for health policy and trauma prevention.

Similarities have been identified between Japan and the Philippines regarding trends, screening, and diagnosis of neurodevelopmental disorders in children (Estrada et al. 2020). In Japan, cases of ADHD and ASD have significantly increased in recent years; for instance, the rate of autism was recorded at 1 in 5000 in 1975 but found to be 1 in 100 in a more recent survey (Weintraub 2011). The Philippines has also reported an increase in ASD cases, rising from 500,000 in 2008 to 1,000,000 in 2018 (Lambatin 2018). Initial identification of neurodevelopmental disorders in both countries is typically conducted in schools, with referrals made to hospitals for diagnosis if cases are identified.

Both Japan and the Philippines have recognized suicide and gaming disorders as major social issues leading to trauma. In the Philippines, common circumstances correlated with mental health concerns among youth include excessive academic pressure and difficulties in time management, compounded by excessive use of digital devices for network gaming and social media. This engagement can lead to depression, a breakdown of personal connections, and cyberbullying. The Philippines, being one of the most active users of social media (Pond et al. 2020), poses a risk for adolescent addiction and depression. In Japan, popular First-Person Shooter (FPS) games also present a dangerous threat to young children (Estrada et al. 2020). Prolonged engagement in these activities may lead to psychological trauma.

During disasters, children and adolescents experience a wide range of mental and behavioural trauma, manifesting as sleeplessness, fear, anxiety, depression, and even post-traumatic stress disorder (Kar 2009). For instance, children affected by the Great East Japan Earthquake (GEJE) experienced long-term sleep disruptions (Usami et al. 2019). Those from the Fukushima area exhibit increasing rates of suicide, child abuse, bullying, and absenteeism, indicating they are among the most affected. Some suicide risks and psychological symptoms have been observed among junior high school students even five years after the disaster. Children who experienced evacuation and temporary housing had externalization symptoms and concerns. Economic disparities, parents' mental health, and a lack of social support also impact these children. Additionally, caring for disabled children after disasters presents challenges, as those with ASD struggle to adjust to crowded evacuation centres (Estrada et al. 2020).

In the Philippines, evacuation centres become very crowded after a disaster, affecting the mental health of children, adolescents, and their families. The lack of mental health services for children is critical, particularly in a country where over 90% of the population identifies as Christian. Religion plays a significant role in the social fabric and has become an important pathway for psychosocial support. Faith-based organizations have established mental health and psychosocial support services (MHPSSs), especially during disasters such as Typhoon Haiyan in 2013 (Final report 2014). Mental health problems can impact children long after disasters (Kar 2009), highlighting the need for mental health support (CDC 2020). After traumatic experiences, schools and, more specifically, school teachers play an essential role in maintaining the well-being of children and adolescents (Mutch 2014). Psychological first aid is described as a "humane, supportive response to a fellow human being who is suffering and who may need support" (WHO 2020a, b). In both Japan and the Philippines, teachers are trained in psychological first aid (PFA) to identify traumatized children and conduct play sessions and storytelling activities to help them cope (Estrada et al. 2020).

In Japan, the most common type of abuse is psychological abuse in younger children (Estrada et al. 2020). Most deaths from abuse are perpetrated by mothers. Neighbours often report cases of child abuse to counselling centres via a 24-hour hotline. Child counselling centres face challenges due to the rapidly increasing cases of post-traumatic stress disorders related to child abuse.

In the Philippines, child abuse manifests through online child sexual exploitation and substance abuse, with the country recognized as one of the top sources of child pornography (UNICEF 2020a). This issue has been reported as an emerging social concern. While an increasing trend in sexual abuse has been observed, physical abuse is likely underreported. Corporal punishment is commonly accepted as a disciplinary method for Filipino children. Surprisingly, psychological abuse is the least recognized and reported form of abuse, despite a national baseline study indicating that 3 of 5 children experience it (UNICEF 2020b). Medical and psychosocial care for abused women and children in the Philippines is provided by the Women and Child Protection Unit (WCPU), utilizing trauma-informed psychosocial processing and cognitive behavioural therapy (CBT) principles to treat affected children.

Definition of Formal Help-Seeking Behaviour

Formal psychological help-seeking behaviour is defined as seeking services and treatment from trained mental healthcare providers, such as psychotherapy and counselling (Rickwood and Thomas 2012). Attitudes toward psychological help-seeking reflect evaluative beliefs about consulting professionals (Divin et al. 2018).

Trauma Exposure and Injury Classification

Understanding trauma exposure is crucial in help-seeking contexts. Patients may describe trauma exposure in terms of injury, which is defined as "physical damage that results when a human body is suddenly or briefly subjected to intolerable levels of energy". Injuries can be classified by their cause (e.g. mechanical, thermal, chemical) or by anatomical location (e.g. head, chest). In the Philippines, common injury categories related to trauma include open wounds, superficial injuries, fractures of the hand, minor traumatic brain injuries, and fractures of the patella, tibia, or fibula (Rivera et al. 2018).

Mental Health Problems Among Children and Adolescents

Globally, an estimated 10–20% of children and adolescents experience mental health problems, with over half of these cases occurring before age 14 (WHO 2020a; Kessler et al. 2007). Mental disorders are the leading cause of disability-adjusted life years (DALYs) among children in the Western Pacific Region (Baranne and Falissard 2018), and the prevalence of suicide attempts is high (Uddin et al. 2019). However, these statistics may be underreported due to the stigma surrounding mental health issues. The WHO's Mental Health Action Plan emphasizes the need for mental health promotion during early life stages (WHO 2020b). While Southeast Asian countries have implemented mental health education focused on coping skills for students, there is a growing interest in creating supportive environments for mental health in schools (Nishio et al. 2020).

Individual Care

There is a critical need for multidisciplinary teams to manage individual cases of trauma (Estrada et al. 2020). These teams may include psychiatrists, social workers, nurses, and occupational therapists. In child abuse cases, nurses and social workers can serve as case managers. These professionals should receive training in various forms of psychotherapy, such as trauma-focused cognitive behavioural therapy (TF-CBT), which is defined as "evidence-based psychotherapy or counselling that aims to address the needs of children and adolescents with post-traumatic stress disorders and other difficulties related to traumatic life events" (de Arellano et al. 2014).

Social Trauma

Social trauma significantly impacts the mental health of an individual and the community as a whole. The pervasive and chronic nature of trauma leads to feelings of despair, hopelessness, and isolation from society. Also, the people unaffected have had to bear the pain of trauma and feel distressed hearing the consequences. Resilience and psychological trauma are interrelated; these complex concepts share similar characteristics (Satapathy et al. 2022). Psychological trauma and resilience are considered products of interaction between individuals, families, and the environment. Trauma at an early age leads to adverse physical, behavioural, and mental health consequences, which can further impair the overall growth and development of an individual in society (Satapathy et al. 2022).

Traumatic experiences or difficult times test an individual; however, the response pattern of each individual varies to different types of traumas. Social support in the form of family, society, and friends helps a person bounce back from the social trauma experiences. Research reported a positive relationship between the availability of social support and resilience. In a study, it has been reported that the availability of a socially supportive environment enhances the resilience to combat bad experiences and trauma (Dar et al. 2021). Resilience in trauma helps in comfortable adaptation and mitigates the adverse effects to allow an individual to behave generally in day-to-day life. Trauma resilience helps an individual alleviate painful experiences and ease the normal grieving process. Resilience is the ability of an individual to adapt and return to psychological homeostasis after going through an unfortunate traumatic event.

Trauma Resilience

Resilience as a personality ingredient is of utmost necessity for humans to survive in the universe. Resilience is the capacity to bounce back or rebound from mental and physical health after traumatic events across the life span. However, resilience trajectories of one individual vary and depend on many factors, including living environment, challenges faced, and individuals' physiologic and genetic makeup (Kaur et al. 2021). Trauma nurses play a pivotal role in the recovery and adaption of individuals, their families, communities, and societies to ameliorate harm.

Role of Nurse in Trauma Resilience

Trauma nurses witness a lot of suffering and injustice with patients who come with different traumas and undergo intervention for life and organ or limb-saving surgeries. Nurses are responsible for supporting the individual and their family or relatives to rebound and return to everyday life. However, trauma nurses should be aware of certain factors that may influence each trauma patient's rebuilding resilience, including environmental context. It has been discussed to view trauma people holistically to choose care based on individual differences, which helps a nurse deliver care that fosters abilities and minimizes difficulties in resilience-building (Tomey and Alligood 2009). Trauma nurses should recognize that humans continuously strive to adjust to the external environment and have their adaptation process during trauma care. The society-to-cells resilience model gives comprehensive coverage of specific nursing theories to understand the role of individual, societal, community, familial, physiological, and cellular factors in resilience development (Szanton and Gill 2010). Understanding that the environment and humans are supplementary to each other will help recognize essential nursing practices to promote adaptation.

Application of the Society-to-Cells Model in Trauma Resilience

The society-to-cells model has six fundamental tenets to understand the process of the resilience of any individual in a specific environment. Details of these six basic tenets of trauma resilience are explained in this chapter. These factors may not be directly related to every trauma victim, and they might interact to create resilience and help to bring the victim to the pre-traumatic stage.

Individual Resilience Potential Each human is born with specific unique resilience potential and tries to resist or bounce back to the pre-trauma stage with full potential. Nurses, while providing trauma care, should keep in mind the genetic or physiological make that can help them bounce back to the pre-trauma stage. For example, females by sex are disadvantaged relative to men historically, and this makes them more vulnerable to sexual- and gender-based violence and hence may need more support to be resilient after trauma (Dar et al. 2021).

Case Study
M.A. is an 80-year-old Thai woman living in a rural province with her five-year-old grandson in a thatched house on someone else's land. After her husband passed away from lung cancer ten years ago, her son abandoned her for a year. M.A. worked as a farmer to support her son through high school and sent him to live with relatives in Bangkok for better job opportunities. After securing a job as a factory worker, her son started a family and asked M.A. to care for his son when he was two months old, promising to send monthly financial support.

M.A. had to quit farming due to health issues, receiving 500 Thai Baht (15 USD) from her son each month, along with 700 Thai Baht (21 USD) from a government pension and 300 Thai Baht (9 USD) from social welfare. Despite this income, it was insufficient for two people's living expenses. Her son declined additional help due to his own financial struggles, and after his marriage ended when the child was five, he cut off support, leaving M.A. responsible for both her and her grandson's needs.

Currently, M.A. suffers from blurry vision and fatigue without prior medical records or access to healthcare due to her remote living situation. She relies on villagers and monks for food. A village health volunteer informed a nurse about M.A.'s situation. During a visit, M.A. expressed her hope for her son to support her in her old age, reflecting her commitment to caring for him as a mother.

Plan of Care

1. *Physical Health Needs*
   M.A.'s physical health issues should be assessed in a healthcare setting, including evaluating her activities of daily living and self-care. If her symptoms are medical, she should receive treatment from primary care and possibly specialty care. Organizations may offer free advanced medical treatment for those in poverty.
2. *Mental Health Needs*
   Assessing M.A.'s mental health can help address potential depression. Collaboration with neighbours, village health volunteers, and religious leaders may encourage M.A. to express her concerns. If she wishes to reconnect with her son, the nurse can assist in facilitating communication.
3. *Healthcare Access*
   M.A. has the right to access basic healthcare through Thailand's universal coverage scheme established in 2022. However, financial constraints and trans-

portation issues may hinder her access. Local government support, community assistance, or volunteer drivers could help her reach healthcare services.

4. *Prepare for Challenges*

Developing a backup plan and resources for M.A. can help her navigate future challenges. Although she receives some government support, it may not be enough for both her and her grandson. The nurse can provide information about job opportunities suitable for the elderly and help set goals for M.A. to improve her situation.

5. *Grandson's Needs*

M.A.'s grandson has also been affected by family adversity. His physical, mental, and social health needs assessment is necessary to ensure he receives adequate nutrition, health screenings, and vaccinations. Additionally, the nurse should evaluate M.A.'s capacity to care for her grandson and assess any potential exposure to domestic violence.

References

Baranne ML, Falissard B (2018) Global burden of mental disorders among children aged 5–14 years. Child Adolesc Psychiatry Ment Health 12(1):Article 19. https://doi.org/10.1186/s13034-018-0225-4

de Arellano MA, Lyman DR, Jobe-Shields L, George P, Dougherty RH, Daniels AS, Ghose SS, Huang L, Delphin-Rittmon ME (2014) Trauma-focused cognitive-behavioral therapy for children and adolescents: assessing the evidence. Psychiatric Services (Washington, D.C.) 65(5):591–602. https://doi.org/10.1176/appi.ps.201300255

Dar AA, Dar S, Deb S, Thomas S, Dhamodharan M, Jahan F, Sumaiya B, Gupta S (2021) Evidence and predictors of resilience among young adults exposed to traumatic events of the armed conflict in Kashmir. Child Youth Serv 42(3):251–273

Divin N, Harper P, Curran E, Corry D, Leavey G (2018) Help-seeking measures and their use in adolescents: a systematic review. Adolesc Res Rev 3:Article 1. https://doi.org/10.1007/s40894-017-0078-8

Earls MF (2018) Trauma-informed primary care: prevention, recognition, and promoting Resilience. N C Med J 79(2):108–112. https://doi.org/10.18043/ncm.79.2.108

Estrada CA, Usami M, Satake N et al (2020) Current situation and challenges for mental health focused on treatment and care in Japan and The Philippines – highlights of the training program by the National Center for Global Health and Medicine. BMC Proc 14(Suppl 11):11. https://doi.org/10.1186/s12919-020-00194-0

Guedes A (2018) Violence against children in Latin America and the Caribbean: data and action. Pan American Health Organization. https://www.paho.org/en/documents/presentationviolence-against-children-latin-america-and-caribbean-data-and-action

Haarr R (2020) Research brief: intimate partner violence in five CARICOM countries—findings from national prevalence surveys on violence against women [Research brief]. UN Women. https://www.unwomen.org/sites/default/files/Headquarters/Attachments/Sections/Library/Publications/2020/Research-brief-Intimate-partner-violence-in-five-CARICOM-countries-en.pdf

Kar N (2009) Psychological impact of disasters on children: review of assessment and interventions. World J Pediatr 5(1):5–11. https://doi.org/10.1007/s12519-009-0001-x

Kaur T, Ranjan P, Chakrawarty A et al (2021) Association of sociodemographic parameters with depression, anxiety, stress, sleep quality, psychological trauma, mental well-being, and resilience during the second wave of COVID-19 pandemic: a cross-sectional survey from India. Cureus 13(7):e16420. https://doi.org/10.7759/cureus.16420

Kessler RC, Angermeyer M, Anthony JC, de Graaf R, Demyttenaere K, Gasquet I, DE Girolamo G, Gluzman S, Gureje O, Haro JM, Kawakami N, Karam A, Levinson D, Medina Mora ME, Oakley Browne MA, Posada-Villa J, Stein DJ, Adley Tsang CH, Aguilar-Gaxiola S, Alonso J et al (2007) Lifetime prevalence and age-of-onset distributions of mental disorders in the World Health Organization's world mental health survey initiative. World Psychiatry 6(3):168–176

Kudva KG, El Hayek S, Gupta AK, Kurokawa S, Bangshan L, Armas-Villavicencio MVC, Oishi K, Mishra S, Tiensuntisook S, Sartorius N (2020) Stigma in mental illness: perspective from eight Asian nations. Asia-Pac Psychiatry 12(2):e12380. https://doi.org/10.1111/appy.12380

Lambatin LO Jr (2018) Persons with autism rising. Philippine Information Agency. https://pia.gov.ph/news/articles/1006481

Maharaj S, Seepersad R, Sooknanan J, Anderson S, Franco D, Ramdass A, Seemungal T (2024) A public health approach to reducing violence within the CARICOM region. Front Public Health 12:1344387. https://doi.org/10.3389/fpubh.2024.1344387

Malee KM, Kerr S, Paul R, Puthanakit T, Thongpibul K, Kosalaraksa P, Ounchanum P, Kanjanavanit S, Aurpibul L, Ngampiyaskul C, Luesomboon W, Wongsawat J, Vonthanak S, Ly PS, Chettra K, Suwanlerk T, Sophonphan J, Valcour V, Ananworanich J, Mellins CA et al (2019) Emotional and behavioral resilience among children with perinatally acquired HIV in Thailand and Cambodia. AIDS (London, England) 33(Suppl 1(Suppl 1)):S17–S27. https://doi.org/10.1097/QAD.0000000000002182

Manasatchakun P, Roxberg Å, Asp M (2018) Conceptions of healthy aging held by relatives of older persons in Isan-Thai culture: a phenomenographic study. J Aging Res 2018:3734645. https://doi.org/10.1155/2018/3734645

Mutch C (2014) The role of schools in disaster preparedness, response and recovery: what can we learn from the literature? Pastor Care Educ 32(1):5–22. https://doi.org/10.1080/02643944.2014.880123

Nishio A, Kakimoto M, Bermardo TMS, Kobayashi J (2020) Current situation and comparison of school mental health in ASEAN countries. Pediatr Int 62(4):438–443. https://doi.org/10.1111/ped.14137

Pond R, Leeding G, Ryan Dubras W-DD (2020) Digital 2020: 3.8 billion people use social media [infographic]. We Are Social. https://wearesocial.com/blog/2020/01/digital-2020-3-8-billion-peopleuse-social-media

Rickwood D, Thomas K (2012) Conceptual measurement framework for help-seeking for mental health problems. Psychol Res Behav Manag 5:173–183. https://doi.org/10.2147/PRBM.S38707

Rivera A, Lam H, Macalino J (2018) Epidemiology of injuries in The Philippines: an analysis of secondary data. Acta Med Philipp 52(2):180–186

Satapathy S, Dang S, Sagar R, Dwivedi SN (2022) Resilience in children and adolescents survived psychologically traumatic life events: a critical review of application of Resilience assessment tools for clinical referral and intervention. Trauma Violence Abuse 23(1):288–300. https://doi.org/10.1177/1524838020939126

Sittichai R, Smith PK (2018) Bullying and cyberbullying in Thailand: coping strategies and relation to age, gender, religion and victim status. J New Approaches Educ Res 7:24–30. https://doi.org/10.7821/naer.2018.1.254

Substance Abuse and Mental Health Services Administration [SAMHSA] (2014) SAMHSA'S concept of trauma and guidance for a trauma-informed approach, HHS publication no. SMA 14-4884. Substance Abuse and Mental Health Services Administration, Rockville. Retrieved from https://store.samhsa.gov/system/files/sma14-4884.pdf

Szanton SL, Gill JM (2010) Facilitating resilience using a society-to-cells framework: a theory of nursing essentials applied to research and practice. ANS Adv Nurs Sci 33(4):329–343. https://doi.org/10.1097/ANS.0b013e3181fb2ea2

Tomey AM, Alligood MR (2009) Nursing theorists and their work, 4th edn. Elsevier, Mosby

Uddin R, Burton NW, Maple M, Khan SR, Khan A (2019) Suicidal ideation, suicide planning, and suicide attempts among adolescents in 59 low-income and middle-income countries: a population-based study. Lancet Child Adolesc Health 3(4):223–233. https://doi.org/10.1016/S2352-4642(18)30403-6

UNICEF (2020a) A systematic literature review of the drivers of violence affecting children in The Philippines [Executive summary]. UNICEF Philippines. https://www.unicef.org/philippines/media/506/file/National%20Baseline%20Study%20on%20Violence%20Against%20 Children%20in%20the%20Philippines:%20Systematic%20literature%20review%20of%

UNICEF (2020b) National baseline study on violence against children: Philippines executive summary. Council for the Welfare of Children & UNICEF Philippines. https://www.unicef.org/philippines/media/491/file/National%20Baseline%20Study%20on%20Violence%20Against%20 Children%20in%20the%20Philippines:%20Results%20(executive%20summary).pdf

Usami M, Iwadare Y, Ushijima H, Inazaki K, Tanaka T, Kodaira M, Watanabe K, Kawahara K, Morikawa M, Kontani K, Murakami K, Ogata R, Okamoto S, Sekine K, Sato M, Sasaki Y, Tanaka H, Harada M, Imagi S, Matsuda K et al (2019) Did kindergarteners who experienced the great East Japan earthquake as infants develop traumatic symptoms? Series of questionnaire-based cross-sectional surveys: a concise and informative title: traumatic symptoms of kindergarteners who experienced disasters as infants. Asian J Psychiatr 44:38–44. https://doi.org/10.1016/j.ajp.2019.07.011

Weintraub K (2011) The prevalence puzzle: autism counts. Nature 479(7371):22–24. https://doi.org/10.1038/479022a

WHO (2020a) Child and adolescent mental health [Internet]. World Health Organization. [cited 2020 Mar 06.]. Available from: https://www.who.int/mental_health/maternalchild/child_adolescent/en/

WHO (2020b) Mental Health Action Plan 2013–2020 [Internet]. World Health Organization; 2013 [cited 2020 Mar 10]. Available from https://apps.who.int/iris/bitstream/handle/10665/89966/9789241506021_eng.pdf;jsessionid=3E09FA457C31F4CAF837E14AD6 FD2B18?sequence=1

Addressing Trauma: Behavioural Outcomes

13

Tamar Rodney

Objectives
- To describe cumulative trauma
- To explore the biopsychosocial effects of cumulative trauma
- To discuss therapeutic challenges and barriers to healing posed by cumulative trauma
- To describe nursing assessment care approaches for individuals with cumulative trauma histories

Introduction

Trauma can profoundly impact an individual's behaviour, often leading to various maladaptive responses that complicate the healing process. Behavioural outcomes stemming from trauma may include increased anxiety, depression, withdrawal from social interactions, and heightened aggression or irritability. These behaviours often manifest an internal struggle, where individuals grapple with feelings of helplessness, fear, and loss of control. Furthermore, trauma can disrupt the neurobiological pathways associated with emotional regulation, leading to difficulties in managing stress and emotions (Laricchiuta et al. 2023). This dysregulation can result in behaviours such as substance abuse or self-harm, which individuals may resort to as coping mechanisms (Weis et al. 2022; Westphal et al. 2017; Zaorska et al. 2020). The cumulative effect of these behaviours can create a cycle that exacerbates the trauma, hindering recovery and impacting the individual's overall quality of life (Hakamata et al. 2022).

T. Rodney (✉)
Johns Hopkins University School of Nursing, Baltimore, MD, USA
e-mail: trodney1@jhu.edu

© The Author(s), under exclusive license to Springer Nature Switzerland AG 2025
T. Rodney (ed.), *Trauma Informed Care*,
https://doi.org/10.1007/978-3-031-87526-7_13

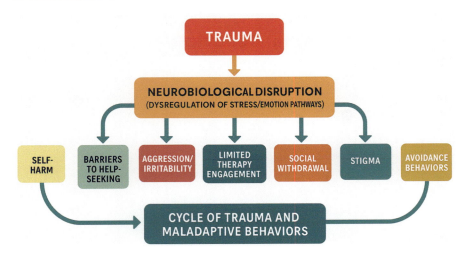

Fig. 13.1 Impact of trauma on behavioural outcomes and healing

The healing process for individuals with trauma histories is often complicated by the interplay of these behavioural outcomes. For many, the journey to recovery is fraught with challenges, as the very behaviours that arise from trauma can serve as barriers to seeking help or engaging in therapeutic interventions. For example, a person exhibiting avoidance behaviours may struggle to attend therapy sessions or share their experiences, limiting their ability to process the trauma (Services 2016). Similarly, the stigma surrounding mental health can prevent individuals from accessing necessary support (Ahad et al. 2023). This creates a significant barrier to healing, as the longer individuals remain trapped in this cycle of trauma and maladaptive behaviours, the more entrenched their conditions may become (Fig. 13.1). Therefore, understanding how trauma manifests in behavioural outcomes is crucial for developing effective healing strategies that address both the psychological and behavioural aspects of recovery (Services 2016).

Cumulative Trauma

Cumulative trauma refers to prolonged exposure to multiple traumatic events, which can include physical, emotional, or psychological harm. Unlike single-event trauma, cumulative trauma often results from a series of stressors that may occur over time, leading to a gradual accumulation of distress (Sacchi et al. 2020). The importance of recognizing cumulative trauma in diverse populations, such as survivors of domestic violence, refugees, and individuals experiencing chronic illness, is pivotal to determining the appropriate treatment. Understanding the complexity of cumulative trauma is essential for healthcare providers to deliver effective interventions that address the unique needs of affected individuals (Han et al. 2021).

Biopsychosocial Effects of Cumulative Trauma

The effects of cumulative trauma can be profound and far-reaching, impacting individuals at biological, psychological, and social levels. Biologically, chronic exposure to trauma can lead to alterations in brain structure and function, including changes in the hypothalamic–pituitary–adrenal (HPA) axis, which regulates stress responses (Cascino and Monteleone 2024; Mbiydzenyuy and Qulu 2024). These changes can manifest as heightened anxiety, depression, and other mental health disorders (Fiksdal et al. 2019). Psychologically, individuals may experience a range of symptoms, including post-traumatic stress disorder (PTSD), anxiety, depression, and difficulties with emotional regulation (Wang et al. 2023). Socially, cumulative trauma can disrupt relationships, lead to social isolation, and diminish an individual's capacity to engage with their community (Services 2016). These interconnected effects help to illustrate how trauma can permeate every aspect of an individual's life and hinder their ability to heal.

Therapeutic Challenges and Barriers to Healing

Therapeutic challenges and barriers to healing are significant factors in the recovery process for individuals with cumulative trauma histories. Mistrust of healthcare providers can arise due to previous negative experiences or systemic discrimination, making it difficult for individuals to engage in treatment (Services 2016). Additionally, the fragmentation of care, often resulting from multiple providers and services, can lead to confusion and disengagement (Joo 2023). By examining these challenges in detail, we can better understand how they manifest in clinical settings and impede therapeutic progress. This exploration can also help identify systemic barriers that contribute to limited access to mental health services. Recognizing these challenges is crucial for healthcare professionals to develop strategies that foster trust and promote effective engagement with individuals affected by trauma.

Nursing Assessment and Care Approaches

Comprehensive nursing assessments are essential for understanding the unique needs of individuals with cumulative trauma histories. A holistic approach to assessment should consider biological, psychological, and social factors (Services 2016). Key components of the assessment include screening for trauma history, identifying co-occurring mental health disorders, and evaluating social support networks (Services 2016). Evidence-based care strategies focus on trauma-informed care principles and should prioritize safety, empowerment, and collaboration (Menschner et al. 2016). These principles create an environment conducive to healing. Mindfulness practices, such as grounding techniques and mindfulness-based stress reduction, serve as effective interventions for promoting emotional regulation and resilience (Gibson 2024; Schuman-Olivier et al. 2020).

Trauma-informed approaches have emerged in response to research demonstrating that trauma is widespread across society, highly correlated with mental health issues, and a costly public health concern. The fundamental shift in providing support using a trauma-informed approach is to move from thinking 'What is wrong with you?' to considering 'What happened to you?' (Sweeney et al. 2018). This reframing emphasizes the need to understand trauma as the cause of mental distress for many service users and the potential for service users to be retraumatized by 'trauma-uninformed' staff. Collaborative care models, which involve interdisciplinary teams, are crucial for addressing the multifaceted needs of individuals affected by trauma. This coordinated approach ensures that all aspects of their well-being are considered and supported throughout their healing journey.

Conclusion

It is critical to understand the importance of cumulative trauma and its impact on behavioural outcomes and the healing process. By recognizing the complex interplay of biological, psychological, and social factors, healthcare professionals can provide more effective, individualized care for those affected by cumulative trauma. The need for trauma-informed approaches in practice is paramount to fostering resilience and promoting recovery. Ultimately, the insights shared in this chapter aim to equip healthcare providers with the knowledge and skills necessary to support individuals on their healing journey, paving the way for improved mental health outcomes and overall well-being.

Case Study

The Impact of Cumulative Trauma on a Young Adult

Tory is a 28-year-old woman who has experienced a series of traumatic events throughout her life. She grew up in a low-income neighbourhood where she was exposed to violence and crime. At the age of 10, she witnessed her father being shot in a gang-related incident. Following this traumatic event, Tory's family faced ongoing financial difficulties, resulting in frequent relocations and instability. During her teenage years, Tory experienced bullying at school, which further impacted her self-esteem. At 18, she suffered a sexual assault, leading to significant psychological distress. Despite these experiences, Tory completed her education and secured a job in marketing. However, she often feels overwhelmed by anxiety, depression, and a sense of hopelessness.

Tory seeks therapy after experiencing a panic attack at work. She reports difficulty concentrating, frequent nightmares related to her past traumas, and a pervasive sense of distrust in others. Tory's relationships are strained; she finds it hard to connect with friends and has withdrawn from social activities she once enjoyed. In therapy, she expresses feelings of inadequacy and struggles to manage her emotions, which she attributes to her cumulative trauma.

Questions

1. As healthcare advocates, how can you recognize and assess the specific traumatic events Tory has experienced, and what signs might indicate that these events are impacting her psychological well-being?
2. Considering Tory's history of cumulative trauma, what challenges might arise in her healing process, and what strategies can you employ to create a supportive and therapeutic environment that acknowledges her trauma?
3. What assessment tools and interventions are effective for evaluating Tory's mental health, and how can you advocate for the incorporation of trauma-informed care principles into her treatment plan to foster resilience and facilitate her recovery?

References

Ahad AA, Sanchez-Gonzalez M, Junquera P (2023) Understanding and addressing mental health stigma across cultures for improving psychiatric care: a narrative review. Cureus 15(5):e39549. https://doi.org/10.7759/cureus.39549

Cascino G, Monteleone AM (2024) Early traumatic experiences and the hypothalamus-pituitary-adrenal axis in people with eating disorders: a narrative review. Psychoneuroendocrinology 159:106665. https://doi.org/10.1016/j.psyneuen.2023.106665

Fiksdal A, Hanlin L, Kuras Y, Gianferante D, Chen X, Thoma MV, Rohleder N (2019) Associations between symptoms of depression and anxiety and cortisol responses to and recovery from acute stress. Psychoneuroendocrinology 102:44–52. https://doi.org/10.1016/j.psyneuen.2018.11.035

Gibson J (2024) Trauma, early life stress, and mindfulness in adulthood. BMC Psychol 12(1):71. https://doi.org/10.1186/s40359-024-01563-6

Hakamata Y, Suzuki Y, Kobashikawa H, Hori H (2022) Neurobiology of early life adversity: a systematic review of meta-analyses towards an integrative account of its neurobiological trajectories to mental disorders. Front Neuroendocrinol 65:100994. https://doi.org/10.1016/j.yfrne.2022.100994

Han HR, Miller HN, Nkimbeng M, Budhathoki C, Mikhael T, Rivers E et al (2021) Trauma informed interventions: a systematic review. PLoS One 16(6):e0252747. https://doi.org/10.1371/journal.pone.0252747

Joo JY (2023) Fragmented care and chronic illness patient outcomes: a systematic review. Nurs Open 10(6):3460–3473. https://doi.org/10.1002/nop2.1607

Laricchiuta D, Panuccio A, Picerni E, Biondo D, Genovesi B, Petrosini L (2023) The body keeps the score: the neurobiological profile of traumatized adolescents. Neurosci Biobehav Rev 145:105033. https://doi.org/10.1016/j.neubiorev.2023.105033

Mbiydzenyuy NE, Qulu LA (2024) Stress, hypothalamic-pituitary-adrenal axis, hypothalamic-pituitary-gonadal axis, and aggression. Metab Brain Dis 39:1613. https://doi.org/10.1007/s11011-024-01393-w

Menschner C, Maul A, Center for Health Care Strategies, I., & Foundation, R. W. J (2016) Key ingredients for successful trauma-informed care implementation. Center for Health Care Strategies, Incorporated

Sacchi L, Merzhvynska M, Augsburger M (2020) Effects of cumulative trauma load on long-term trajectories of life satisfaction and health in a population-based study. BMC Public Health 20(1):1612. https://doi.org/10.1186/s12889-020-09663-9

Schuman-Olivier Z, Trombka M, Lovas DA, Brewer JA, Vago DR, Gawande R et al (2020) Mindfulness and behavior change. Harv Rev Psychiatry 28(6):371–394. https://doi.org/10.1097/hrp.0000000000000277

Services, U. S. D. H. H (2016) A treatment improvement protocol – trauma-informed care in behavioral health services – tip 57. Lulu.com

Sweeney A, Filson B, Kennedy A, Collinson L, Gillard S (2018) A paradigm shift: relationships in trauma-informed mental health services. BJPsych Adv 24(5):319–333. https://doi.org/10.1192/bja.2018.29

Wang SK, Feng M, Fang Y, Lv L, Sun GL, Yang SL et al (2023) Psychological trauma, post-traumatic stress disorder and trauma-related depression: a mini-review. World J Psychiatry 13(6):331–339. https://doi.org/10.5498/wjp.v13.i6.331

Weis CN, Webb EK, deRoon-Cassini TA, Larson CL (2022) Emotion dysregulation following trauma: shared neurocircuitry of traumatic brain injury and trauma-related psychiatric disorders. Biol Psychiatry 91(5):470–477. https://doi.org/10.1016/j.biopsych.2021.07.023

Westphal M, Aldao A, Jackson C (2017) Emotion dysregulation in comorbid posttraumatic stress disorder and substance use disorders: a narrative review. Mil Psychol 29:216. https://doi.org/10.1037/mil0000157

Zaorska J, Kopera M, Trucco EM, Suszek H, Kobyliński P, Jakubczyk A (2020) Childhood trauma, emotion regulation, and pain in individuals with alcohol use disorder. Front Psych 11:554150. https://doi.org/10.3389/fpsyt.2020.554150

Addressing Trauma: Reshaping the Future

14

Chitchanok Benjasirisan, Pearl Ed Cuevas, Veroina Deslandes, Louise Isham, Suratsawadee Kruahong, Rajesh Kumar, Emma Mangano, Eugenia Millender, Georgina Morley, Michelle Patch, Tamar Rodney, Thitipong Tankampuan, and Patty Wilson

Objectives
- Understand the principles of trauma-informed care to recognize its significance in patient recovery and support
- Apply trauma-informed care knowledge by integrating relevant topics into nursing coursework and clinical training
- Analyse assessment strategies and design a timeline for ongoing patient evaluations that address the evolving nature of trauma recovery

---

C. Benjasirisan · S. Kruahong · E. Mangano · M. Patch · T. Rodney (✉) · P. Wilson
Johns Hopkins University School of Nursing, Baltimore, MD, USA
e-mail: trodney1@jhu.edu

P. E. Cuevas
Centro Escolar University Manila, Manila, Philippines

V. Deslandes
University of the West Indies-Mona, Kingston, Jamaica

L. Isham
Department of Social Work and Social Care, University of Birmingham, Birmingham, UK

R. Kumar
All India Institute of Medical Sciences, Rishikesh, Uttarakhand, India

E. Millender
Florida State University, Tallahassee, FL, USA

G. Morley
Center for Bioethics & Stanley S. Zielony Institute for Nursing Excellence, Cleveland Clinic, Cleveland, OH, USA

T. Tankampuan
Mahidol University Faculty of Nursing, Bangkok, Thailand

© The Author(s), under exclusive license to Springer Nature Switzerland AG 2025
T. Rodney (ed.), *Trauma Informed Care*,
https://doi.org/10.1007/978-3-031-87526-7_14

Introduction

The concept of "dose-related response" in trauma refers to the cumulative effects of trauma exposure over time, impacting individuals differently based on the frequency, duration, and intensity of traumatic experiences. This model helps in understanding how repeated or prolonged trauma can exacerbate physical and mental health challenges, leading to a range of complex, long-lasting effects. A crucial aspect of this response is the timeline of trauma experiences, encompassing intergenerational trauma, collective trauma, and personal histories, all of which influence how trauma manifests across generations. See Table 14.1.

Table 14.1 Description of trauma and nursing implications

Type of trauma	Description	Nursing implications
Intergenerational trauma	Trauma effects are passed from one generation to the next, often seen in descendants with increased anxiety or stress.	Recognize that patients may display trauma symptoms linked to family history, allowing for compassionate, personalized care.
Collective and historical trauma	Trauma impacts entire communities, creating lasting legacies, as seen with descendants of enslaved people who may distrust healthcare systems.	Provide culturally sensitive care by acknowledging historical traumas and addressing patients' unique needs, particularly in marginalized communities.
Transgenerational trauma	Trauma responses pass down through behaviours and biology, with descendants potentially inheriting stress responses, such as those in children of trauma survivors.	Recognize and validate inherited trauma responses, offering care that supports patients dealing with stress linked to ancestral trauma.
Multigenerational trauma	Trauma compounds over generations, as each person faces the original trauma and unresolved responses seen in Indigenous communities affected by colonization.	Address trauma at both individual and family levels, offering a holistic approach that acknowledges the compounded adversity faced by marginalized groups.
Cross-generational trauma	Trauma effects spread indirectly through learned behaviours, attitudes, and cultural narratives, such as mistrust passed down in communities facing systemic racism.	Understand complex patient reactions rooted in shared history, fostering care that considers collective memory and family dynamics.

Dose-Related Responses Over Time

The dose-response model suggests that repeated trauma exposure can amplify the risk of adverse health outcomes, such as PTSD, cardiovascular disease, and substance abuse. Nurses must recognize that patients with a history of repeated trauma, whether through domestic violence, systemic oppression, or socioeconomic hardship, may have an intensified response to current stressors. This cumulative impact of trauma emphasizes the need for trauma-informed care approaches that include detailed assessments, allowing nurses to identify patterns in a patient's trauma history and customize care to support resilience and recovery. By understanding these timeline experiences, nurses can better support patients dealing with the multi-layered impact of trauma. Integrating these insights into trauma-informed care models promotes holistic healing and helps to break cycles of trauma that span generations, ultimately contributing to more equitable health outcomes across diverse populations (see Fig. 14.1).

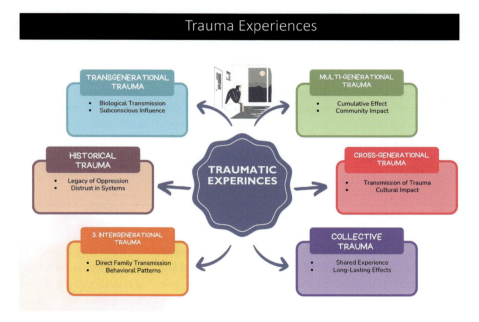

Fig. 14.1 Trauma experiences

Historical Context of Trauma

Trauma manifests uniquely within various historical and collective experiences, each shaped by its specific context and impacting individuals and communities on multiple levels. Understanding these nuanced experiences of trauma is vital in trauma-informed care (TIC), as it allows healthcare professionals to approach each patient with empathy, respect for their history, and a culturally sensitive lens. The importance of TIC is underscored by the need to recognize how trauma influences health outcomes and patient interactions, which is essential for effective healthcare delivery (Ervin et al. 2021; Fleishman et al. 2019; Guest 2021).

Pandemic Trauma

The COVID-19 pandemic represents a recent form of collective trauma that has affected individuals and communities globally. The sudden, pervasive fear of infection, social isolation, loss of loved ones, and economic instability triggered widespread anxiety, depression, and post-traumatic stress symptoms (Grabbe et al. 2021). For healthcare workers, the trauma of managing the crisis with limited resources and high patient mortality rates led to burnout, moral injury, and a lasting impact on mental health (Emsley et al. 2022; Grabbe et al. 2021). Nurses and healthcare providers should consider these pandemic-related experiences, as patients may exhibit residual trauma responses, especially when discussing health-related concerns. Acknowledging the pandemic's impact allows healthcare providers to approach care more sensitively, understanding that even routine medical experiences may trigger pandemic-related anxieties (Emsley et al. 2022; Grabbe et al. 2021).

Trauma Among Holocaust Survivors

Holocaust survivors endured extreme and prolonged trauma, including imprisonment, starvation, the loss of family members, and the constant threat of death. This deeply traumatic experience has left many survivors with symptoms of PTSD, depression, and anxiety, which often persist throughout their lives (Forstmeier et al. 2020; Weissberger et al. 2024). Research indicates that the trauma experienced by Holocaust survivors has a significant intergenerational impact, with descendants sometimes showing higher vulnerability to stress and mental health disorders (Forstmeier et al. 2023; Payne and Berle 2021). Nurses working with Holocaust survivors or their descendants must understand these specific traumas and be prepared to provide care that honours the historical and personal context of their experiences. This sensitivity can help build trust and create a safe space for healing (Forstmeier et al. 2020; Payne and Berle 2021; Weissberger et al. 2024).

Collective Memory and Historical Trauma

Collective memory refers to the shared recollections of traumatic events within a group, often passed down through stories, traditions, and cultural narratives. This concept is especially relevant to communities that have experienced traumatic events as a group, such as Indigenous populations affected by colonization and forced relocation or communities affected by systemic racism (Emsley et al. 2022; Guest 2021). The lasting effects of these traumas shape group identity and influence individuals' perceptions and responses to current stressors.

Nurses should be aware of these shared histories, as patients may carry the emotional weight of collective trauma, affecting their health, sense of safety, and trust in institutions (Emsley et al. 2022; Guest 2021). Trauma-informed care that respects and acknowledges these histories can help bridge care gaps and foster a more supportive therapeutic relationship (Ervin et al. 2021; Fleishman et al. 2019).

The Trauma of Slavery

The trauma of slavery continues to impact the African American community, both in terms of direct generational effects and through the legacy of systemic racial oppression. Enslaved individuals experienced physical violence, separation from families, dehumanization, and a total lack of autonomy (Emsley et al. 2022; Guest 2021). This historical trauma persists in the form of social and economic disparities, as well as psychological impacts that manifest across generations (Emsley et al. 2022). The effects of slavery contribute to higher rates of chronic stress, mistrust in healthcare, and mental health conditions within African American communities (Guest 2021). Trauma-informed care should, therefore, include an understanding of this historical trauma and its lingering impact, incorporating culturally respectful practices and building trust to mitigate the barriers created by this legacy (Emsley et al. 2022; Guest 2021).

The Future of Trauma-Informed Care

The future of trauma-informed care (TIC) in nursing holds significant promise for enhancing the quality of care provided to individuals with a history of trauma. As the understanding of trauma and its effects on health continues to evolve, several critical components must be acknowledged to advance nursing practice in this area.

Education

Continuous education is key to ensuring that healthcare professionals, particularly nurses, are equipped with the knowledge and skills necessary to support trauma survivors effectively. Continuous education programmes should encompass trauma-informed principles, recognition of trauma symptoms, and patient-centred care approaches. Recent studies emphasize the positive impact of trauma-informed care training on healthcare providers' attitudes and practices, highlighting the necessity for ongoing professional development in this field (Dowdell and Speck 2022; Wholeben et al. 2023; Çınar Özbay et al. 2023).

Inclusion in Nursing Curriculum

Trauma-informed care principles should be integrated into nursing education at all levels. Nursing schools must incorporate trauma-related topics, assessment techniques, and evidence-based interventions into their curricula to prepare future nurses for the complexities of trauma care (Goddard et al. 2022; Kaur et al. 2021; Wholeben et al. 2023). This foundational knowledge is critical for fostering a workforce that is sensitive to the needs of trauma survivors.

Practice

Implementing trauma-informed practices in clinical settings is essential and should reflect trauma-informed principles. Nurses are tasked with creating safe environments, practicing patient-centred communication, and engaging in shared decision-making with trauma survivors. Implementing trauma-informed practices can lead to improved patient outcomes and satisfaction, as evidenced by recent analyses of trauma patient experiences (Watts et al. 2021; Xiang et al. 2022).

Assessment Timeline

Trauma assessment should be dynamic and ongoing, recognizing that individuals may not disclose traumatic experiences immediately. Utilizing trauma screening tools during routine assessments is essential, as is remaining vigilant for signs of trauma-related distress (Chowdhury et al. 2022; Karanikola et al. 2022). Early identification and intervention are crucial; nurses should provide immediate support, validate experiences, and connect patients to appropriate resources for further evaluation and treatment (Goddard et al. 2022).

Polytrauma Management

This is particularly relevant as many individuals with trauma histories may have experienced multiple traumas. Nurses must be skilled in managing complex presentations and addressing the interconnected effects of various traumatic experiences (Kaur et al. 2021; Kim et al. 2023). This requires a comprehensive understanding of trauma's multifaceted nature and its implications for patient care.

Research

Continued research remains essential to expand knowledge about trauma, its impact on health, and effective interventions. Continued investigation into trauma-focused therapies and evidence-based practices will guide nursing care and inform best practices (Wang et al. 2022). Collaborative work among healthcare disciplines, community organizations, and trauma survivors themselves is fundamental in developing comprehensive care models that address the diverse needs of trauma survivors (Karanikola et al. 2022).

Ethical Consideration

Nurses must be mindful of ethical considerations when working with trauma survivors. This must include ensuring there is informed consent, respecting autonomy, and maintaining confidentiality throughout the care process (Dowdell and Speck 2022; Wholeben et al. 2023). Additionally, understanding the long-term impact of trauma, including dose-related responses to cumulative trauma exposures, will inform tailored interventions and long-term care plans (Goddard et al. 2022; Kaur et al. 2021).

Contextual Considerations

Acknowledging the impact of historical traumas, such as the Holocaust and slavery, can deepen nurses' cultural awareness and sensitivity, enhancing their ability to provide trauma-informed care (Goddard et al. 2022; Wholeben et al. 2023). Furthermore, recognizing the traumatic impact of pandemics, such as COVID-19, is crucial in addressing mental health and healthcare disparities among affected populations (Crowe et al. 2021; Karanikola et al. 2022). In conclusion, the future of trauma-informed care in nursing lies in the integration of these critical components into practice, education, and research. By continually advancing trauma-informed approaches, nursing care can play a transformative role in supporting individuals with trauma histories on their journey toward healing, resilience, and overall well-being.

Summary

The future of trauma-informed care lies in the integration of these critical components into nursing practice, education, and research. By continually advancing trauma-informed approaches, nursing care can play a transformative role in supporting individuals with trauma histories on their journey towards healing, resilience, and overall well-being.

Discussion Question

How can you integrate key components of trauma-informed care into your nursing practice to improve outcomes for individuals with a trauma history?

References

Chowdhury S, Almarhabi M, Varghese B, Leenen L (2022) Trauma resuscitation training: an evaluation of nurses' knowledge. J Trauma Nurs 29(4):192–200. https://doi.org/10.1097/jtn.0000000000000661

Crowe S, Howard AF, Vanderspank-Wright B, Gillis P, McLeod F, Penner C, Haljan G (2021) The effect of COVID-19 pandemic on the mental health of Canadian critical care nurses providing patient care during the early phase pandemic: a mixed method study. Intensive Crit Care Nurs 63:102999. https://doi.org/10.1016/j.iccn.2020.102999

Dowdell EB, Speck PM (2022) CE: trauma-informed care in nursing practice. Am J Nurs 122(4):30–38. https://doi.org/10.1097/01.NAJ.0000827328.25341.1f

Emsley E, Smith J, Martin D, Lewis NV (2022) Trauma-informed care in the UK: where are we? A qualitative study of health policies and professional perspectives. BMC Health Serv Res 22(1):1164. https://doi.org/10.1186/s12913-022-08461-w

Ervin K, Reid C, Podubinski T, Phillips J (2021) Trauma-informed knowledge, awareness, practice, competence and confidence of rural health staff: a descriptive study. J Nurs Educ Pract 11:1–8. https://doi.org/10.5430/jnep.v11n9p1

Fleishman JP, Kamsky HBSNRNC, Sundborg SP (2019) Trauma-informed nursing practice. Online J Issues Nurs 24(2):1–9. https://doi.org/10.3912/OJIN.Vol24No02Man03

Forstmeier S, van der Hal E, Auerbach M, Maercker A, Brom D (2020) Life review therapy for holocaust survivors (LRT-HS): study protocol for a randomised controlled trial. BMC Psychiatry 20(1):186. https://doi.org/10.1186/s12888-020-02600-5

Forstmeier S, Zimmermann S, van der Hal E, Auerbach M, Kleinke K, Maercker A, Brom D (2023) Effect of life review therapy for holocaust survivors: a randomized controlled trial. J Trauma Stress 36(3):628–641. https://doi.org/10.1002/jts.22933

Goddard A, Janicek E, Etcher L (2022) Trauma-informed care for the pediatric nurse. J Pediatr Nurs 62:1–9. https://doi.org/10.1016/j.pedn.2021.11.003

Grabbe L, Higgins MK, Baird M, Pfeiffer KM (2021) Impact of a resiliency training to support the mental well-being of front-line workers: brief report of a quasi-experimental study of the community resiliency model. Med Care 59(7):616–621. https://doi.org/10.1097/mlr.0000000000001535

Guest H (2021) A concept analysis of trauma-informed care. Nurs Forum 56(4):1000–1007. https://doi.org/10.1111/nuf.12626

Karanikola M, Mpouzika M, Papathanassoglou E, Kaikoushi K, Hatzioannou A, Leontiou I et al (2022) Work-related traumatic stress response in nurses employed in COVID-19 settings. Int J Environ Res Public Health 19(17). https://doi.org/10.3390/ijerph191711049

Kaur S, Rattan A, Kumar H, Rao S, Kant R, Misra MC (2021) Advanced trauma care for nurses (ATCN): a single-center analysis of trauma nurses knowledge gaps. J Trauma Nurs 28(4):258–264. https://doi.org/10.1097/jtn.0000000000000594

Kim S, Kim GU, Park J (2023) Evaluation of internet-based training in trauma care for nurses in mental health welfare centers: a cluster randomized controlled trial. J Prim Care Community Health 14:21501319231181982. https://doi.org/10.1177/21501319231181982

Payne EA, Berle D (2021) Posttraumatic stress disorder symptoms among offspring of Holocaust survivors: a systematic review and meta-analysis. Traumatology 27(3):254–264. https://doi.org/10.1037/trm0000269

Wang L, Zhang X, Zhang P, Zhou Q, Wang Q, Cheng J (2022) Development and psychometric evaluation of the trauma nurse core competency scale. Front Public Health 10:959176. https://doi.org/10.3389/fpubh.2022.959176

Watts DD, Slivinski A, Garland JM, Kerley DR, Wilson NY, Cooper T et al (2021) The impact of nursing on trauma patient satisfaction: an analysis of HCAHPS from 112,283 patients. J Trauma Nurs 28(4):219–227. https://doi.org/10.1097/jtn.0000000000000589

Weissberger GH, Bensimon M, Shrira A (2024) Financial exploitation and mental health among Holocaust survivors: the moderating role of posttraumatic symptoms. Int Psychogeriatr 36:772. https://doi.org/10.1017/s1041610223000625

Wholeben M, Castro Y, Salazar G, Field C (2023) Impact of trauma-informed care training on attitudes among emergency department personnel, staff advocates, and nursing students. J Trauma Nurs 30(5):261–270. https://doi.org/10.1097/jtn.0000000000000740

Xiang S, Tang W, Shang X, Ni H (2022) Practice of multidisciplinary collaborative chain management model in constructing nursing path for acute trauma treatment. Emerg Med Int 2022:1342773. https://doi.org/10.1155/2022/1342773

Çınar Özbay S, Boztepe H, Kanbay Y (2023) Nursing students' views on trauma-informed pediatric nursing care and family-centered care. Arch Psychiatr Nurs 44:107–113. https://doi.org/10.1016/j.apnu.2023.04.012

Printed in the United States
by Baker & Taylor Publisher Services